William NEALY

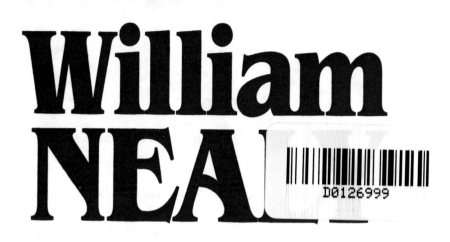

D0126999

Mountain BIKE!

A Manual of Beginning to Advanced Technique

Warning!

This book contains information and techniques that can cause severe damage to the environment, to others, and to yourself.

Damage to the Environment: Some will criticize this book with its descriptions of dyno-moves, skid turns, pivot turns, etc., as being irresponsible and even dangerous to the sport of mountain biking. Everyone loves the racers, the embodiment of dynamic riding, but some feel we shouldn't teach beginners to be too dynamic because they'll automatically abuse the environment. The problem of slob riders mutilating trails is not a matter of too much information, it's a behavior problem. Some places can be ridden wildly (active timbering areas, race courses, powerlines) while some shouldn't be ridden at all (most trails on rainy days, designated wilderness areas, etc.) It's up to the individual rider to learn the difference and ride accordingly. Environmental awareness, safety and courtesy should always be your prime consideration in this decision.

Damage to Others and Yourself: Fun Hogs wilding on high-speed metal contraptions across irregular terrain create a recipe for danger if ever there was one. Each rider must recognize the danger inherent in the sport and accept responsibility for his/her actions on a mountain bike. As for self-inflicted injuries, it all boils down to simple physics: the faster you go, the harder you hit. The rider alone controls the severity of any crash. Remember...Gravity: It isn't just a good idea; it's the law.

Distributed by VELONEWSBOOKS
1830 North 55th Street
Boulder, CO 80301
(303) 440-0601

Library of Congress Cataloging-in-Publication Data
Nealy, William, 1953-
Mountain bike: a manual of technique / by William Nealy
p. cm.
ISBN 0-89732-114-6
1. All terrain cycling. I. Title.
GV1056.N43   1991   91-40292
796.6-dc20   CIP

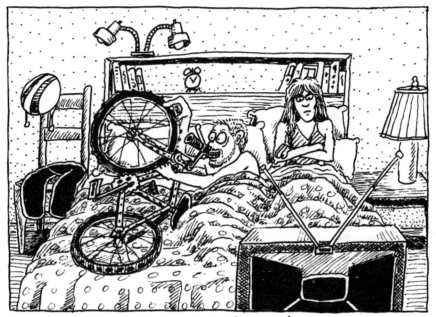

This book is dedicated to Holly,
who loves me anyway...

Acknowledgments

For their significant contributions to mountain bike technique and humor, special thanks to Bruce Tiller, Bob Sehlinger, James Torrence, Johnny Cake, David Vernon, Gordon Sumerel, Madison Torrence, Henry Unger, Tom Schlinkert, Lynn Brandon, Barrie Wallace, John Barbour, Dave Schmidt, David Tanner, Daniel Wallace, Mark Zwick, Tim Blumenthal, Wayne Bob Colwell, Cliff Earle, Mike Jones and everyone at N.O.C.!

Believe me! The secret of reaping the greatest fruitfulness and the greatest enjoyment from life is to live dangerously.

Nietzsche

Table Of Contents

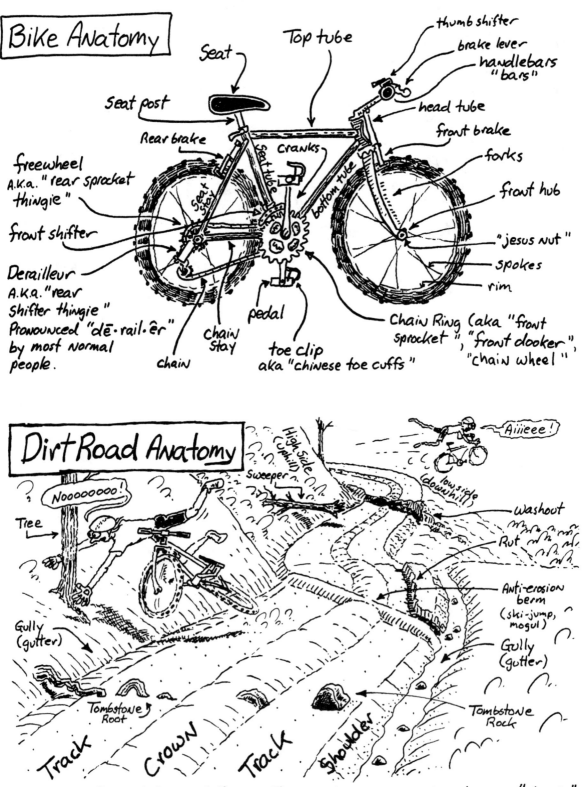

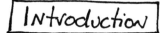

Introduction

This book is an attempt to make advanced riding skills more accessible to the general mountain bike-riding population. Mountain biking is an inherently fun thing to do and it's also a fun thing to learn to do. In fact, the essence of mountain biking is "learning to do", not just doing. To entry-level and novice mtn. bikers, what follows in this book may seem incredibly complex and bewildering. The truth of the matter is: if you ride a <u>lot</u> and never read a word about it, you'll learn to ride a mountain bike well by osmosis given sufficient on-trail experience. This book, hopefully, may provide a few shortcuts on the mountain bike learning curve. The most important thing is to RIDE!

Mountain Biking is simple! To prove it, below is an ultra-refined synopsis of this entire book...

① Ride gently.
② Focus your weight on your feet, not the seat.
③ Use your whole body to propel the bike.
④ Use your gears.
⑤ Keep your bike well-maintained.
⑥ Wear a helmet.
⑦ Ride ride ride!

2

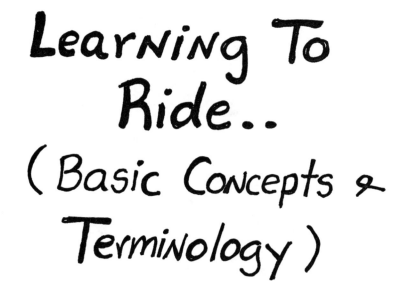

Learning To Ride...
(Basic Concepts & Terminology)

Learning To Learn

Most mtn. bike learning is of the self-instructed experiential variety. To wit, you ride progressively harder & harder stuff, wipe out a lot and learn from your mistakes (see below).

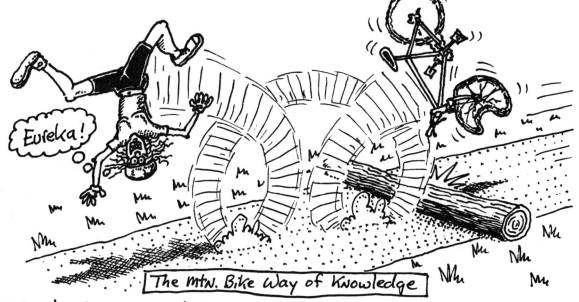

The mtn. Bike Way of Knowledge

Eventually you will train your body to react quickly and instinctively to a wide variety of obstacles and trail conditions while having loads of fun. Mountain biking is a never-ending learning process and as long as you're having fun you are on the learning curve (see below).

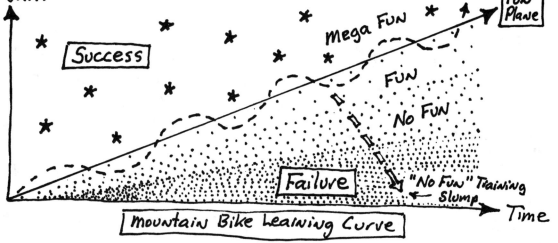

Mountain Bike Learning Curve

The golden rule of successful self-teaching is "Be Kind To Your Student!" Becoming your own Nazi Drill Instructor turns the learning process into work. Once you remove fun from the process you start down the slippery slope of reinforced failure and "learning regression."

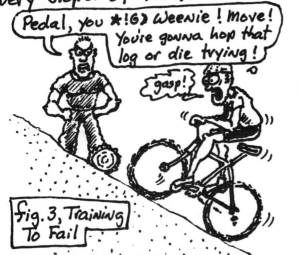

Pedal, you *!6) weenie! move! You're gonna hop that log or die trying!

gasp!

fig. 3, Training To Fail

So, before you begin a self-training session RELAX, this ain't Wall Street. You can't lose riding a mtn. bike.

If you are working on a technique and you fail two or three times in a row, STOP!! Do something else & try again later. This is called "Training To Failure."* If you push a training session beyond three successive failures you are "Training To Fail."* As you become more adept at self-teaching and pushing yourself appropriately you'll be able to discern where good (beneficial) training ends and bad (regressive) training begins. [Hint: lack of fun marks the spot.]

Tailor training sessions to your ability. If your buddies are floating over 18" diameter logs but you're wiping out on 6" logs, Don't throw yourself repeatedly at 18" logs! Start with logs you can do & work your way up incrementally (example: 4" logs then 6" logs then 8" logs, etc.). You'll find that once you've mastered the basic small log hop, successive diameters will have become a problem of amplification [applying more & more power to your hop] not a problem of fundamental technique.

Philosophical Focus Point I: To eat a whole elephant take many small bites and learn to love leftovers.

Philosophical Focus Point II: You can't spell "Fundamental" without "Fun."

_____

*Training To Failure - positive progressive training; pushing the envelope.

*Training To Fail - negative regressive training; more pain than fun.

Instinctualizing Riding Skills...

The **Mountain Bike Cartoon Learning Theory** states that all acquired (learned) riding skills are essentially "**body knowledge**" evolved via experience from "**brain knowledge**". In other words, as a rider gains trail competence & moves up the skill ladder from Novice to expert, he/she is unconsciously converting mental constructs (skills) into instinctive responses by **skill repetition** (practice, training, experience). You can speed up the skill instinctualization process by making it a conscious experience and **Training To Failure** in a fun-oriented context.

Further, all potential mtn. bikers are created **UNEQUAL**! If you happen to be a "body genius"* like Michael Jordan you'll be bunny-hopping transit buses within fifteen min-

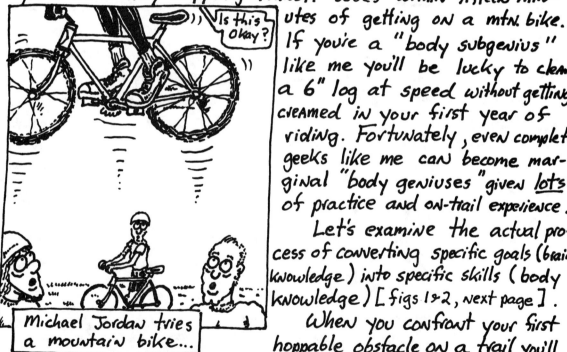

Is this okay?

Michael Jordan tries a mountain bike...

utes of getting on a mtn. bike. If you're a "body subgenius" like me you'll be lucky to clear a 6" log at speed without getting creamed in your first year of riding. Fortunately, even complete geeks like me can become marginal "body geniuses" given _lots_ of practice and on-trail experience.

Let's examine the actual process of converting specific goals (brain knowledge) into specific skills (body knowledge) [figs 1&2, next page].

When you confront your first hoppable obstacle on a trail you'll probably go thru a fairly common mental/physical stimulus → analysis → response cycle: your eyes see the obstacle and tell your brain about it. Your brain analyzes velocity, height of obstacle, etc. and commands the body to react a certain

* "body genius" - athletically gifted. This term does not imply that a so-called "body genius" can't also be a "mental genius".

way to theoretically overcome the obstacle (fig. 1). The problem

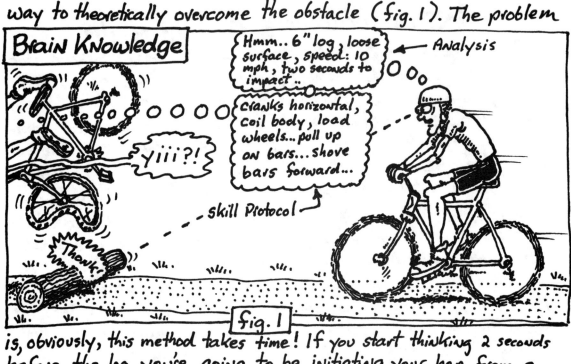

fig. 1

is, obviously, this method takes time! If you start thinking 2 seconds before the log, you're going to be initiating your hop from a prone position 10 feet past the log, if you're not knocked out in the crash. Clearly, thinking (analysis) has to be virtually eliminated from the stimulus→response cycle. The trick is to create a log-hopping protocol and train it in until it is internalized & instinctive. One approach to this learning situation would be to stop, think through the necessary moves, then have a go at the log at a slower-than-normal

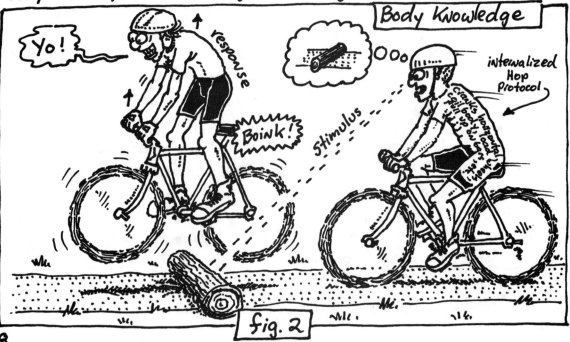

fig. 2

velocity. Keep doing it until ⓐ you're hopping the log perfectly each time at speed, ⓑ you fail two or three consecutive times [Training To Failure], or ⓒ you stop having fun. By stopping **before** frustration sets in and doing something else you avoid mental blocks and keep the experience fresh. If you apply this rational learning process to each biking challenge you'll educate your body quickly and effectively and have loads of fun along the way!

How your mind perceives an obstacle after more than three consecutive failures...

gasp!

Aiiieee!

MTN. Bike Learning
Process focus points:
   1. Stop & formulate a plan.
   2. Make the challenge appropriate and incremental.
   3. Execute the plan to ⓐ Success (yo!)
                         ⓑ Failure (three consecutive failures)'
   4. Analyze the failure & move on to something else.
   5. Have FUN !!

' Further Notes on "Training To Failure" - To keep growing in the sport you've got to learn to push your skill envelope while avoiding serious injury and/or terminal frustration (mental block(s)). Thus, training to failure is NOT training to exhaustion/frustration/psychic destruction. I'm talking about a healthy dialectical tension between your existing skill level and your potential skill level (tempered, of course, by moderation). For example, I'm a fairly inept trials rider but I enjoy trying the occasional trials trail to test existing skills and perhaps learn something new. Any rider can continually challenge himself/herself by riding a little faster and jumping a little higher. As long as the challenges are incremental and limited to two or three failures per challenge, the rider remains on the fun plane and gets better and better. Keep in mind this is all one dude's opinion and what works for me may not work for you. This is but one of many paths to mountain bike Nirvana.

Comparative Psychoanatomy 101

Typical Novice Type

lift bars, cranks horizontal, right pedal stroke, etc

Linear analytical thinking; body responding to mental "commands"

Mind Smart

Focused on immediate obstacle (therefore not anticipating the next successive moves)

sitting on seat, body neutral

Motion slow, moves choppy & exaggerated

Negative Visualization

Typical Honed-To-The-Bone Expert Type

off seat, whole body in "ready mode"

Reacting instinctively (body acting directly on visual information)

Thinking three moves ahead

Focused out to event horizon, anticipating several moves beyond the immediate obstacle.

Motion fast and fluid; minimalist

Event Horizon

yay-hoo!

Positive Visualization

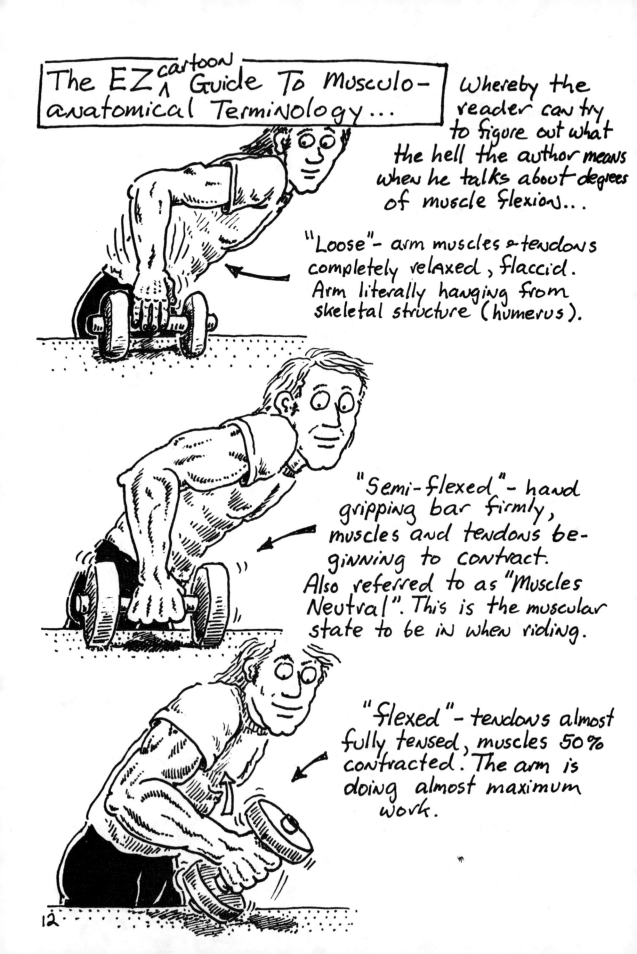

The EZ ^cartoon Guide To Musculo-anatomical Terminology...

Whereby the reader can try to figure out what the hell the author means when he talks about degrees of muscle flexion...

"Loose" - arm muscles & tendons completely relaxed, flaccid. Arm literally hanging from skeletal structure (humerus).

"Semi-flexed" - hand gripping bar firmly, muscles and tendons beginning to contract. Also referred to as "Muscles Neutral". This is the muscular state to be in when riding.

"Flexed" - tendons almost fully tensed, muscles 50% contracted. The arm is doing almost maximum work.

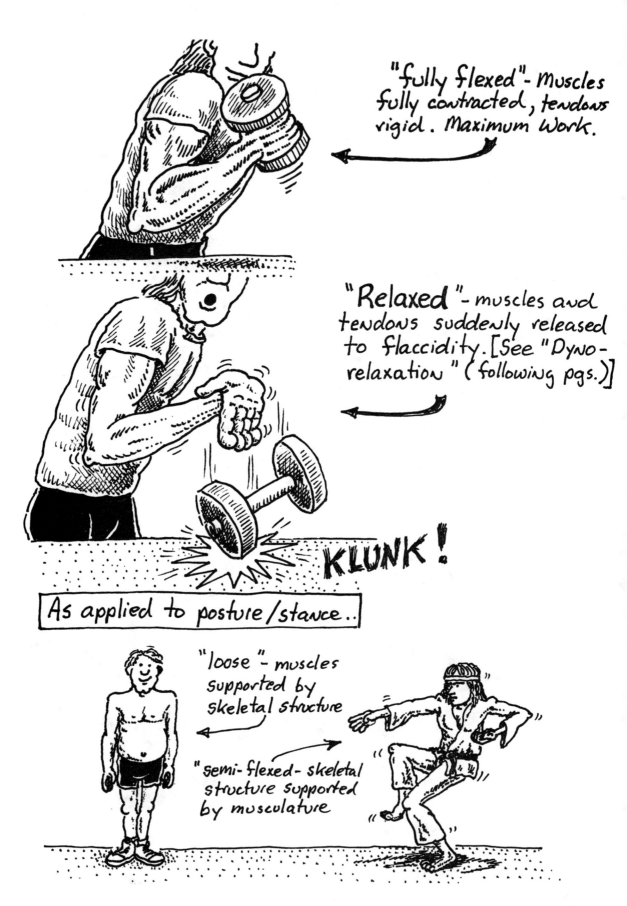

"fully flexed"- Muscles fully contracted, tendons rigid. Maximum Work.

"Relaxed"- muscles and tendons suddenly released to flaccidity. [See "Dyno-relaxation" (following pgs.)]

KLUNK!

As applied to posture/stance..

"loose"- muscles supported by skeletal structure

"semi-flexed- skeletal structure supported by musculature

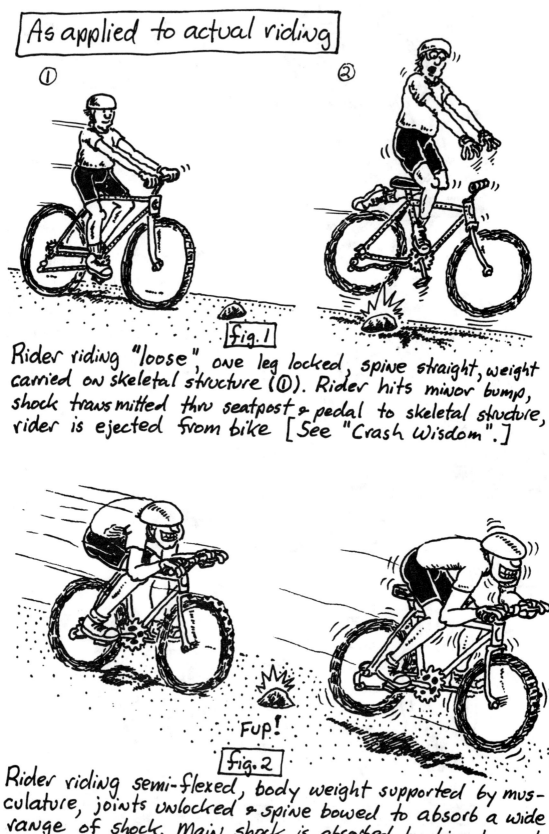

As applied to actual riding

① ②

fig. 1

Rider riding "loose", one leg locked, spine straight, weight carried on skeletal structure (①). Rider hits minor bump, shock transmitted thru seatpost & pedal to skeletal structure, rider is ejected from bike [See "Crash Wisdom".]

FUP!

fig. 2

Rider riding semi-flexed, body weight supported by musculature, joints unlocked & spine bowed to absorb a wide range of shock. Main shock is absorbed by biggest muscles (legs) because rider's weight is focused on pedals...

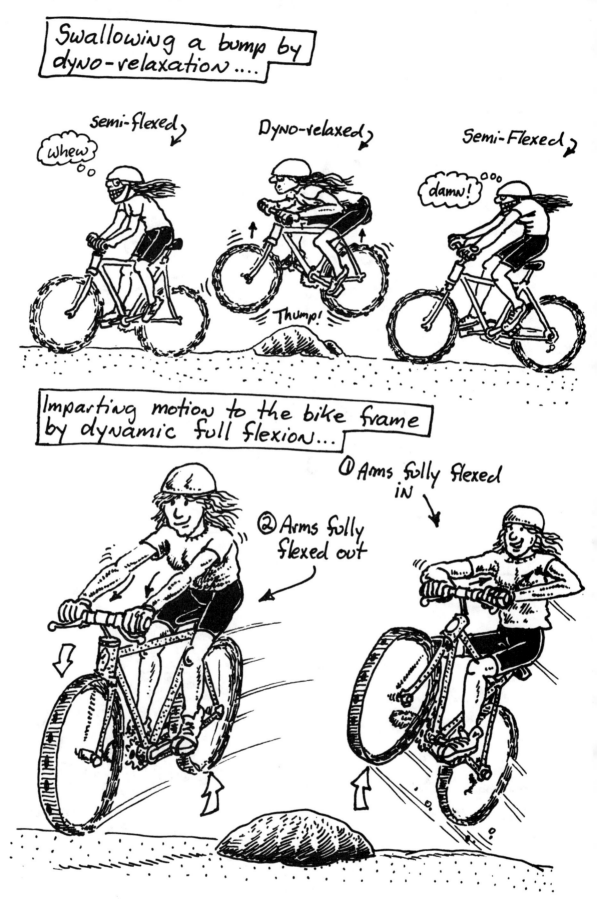

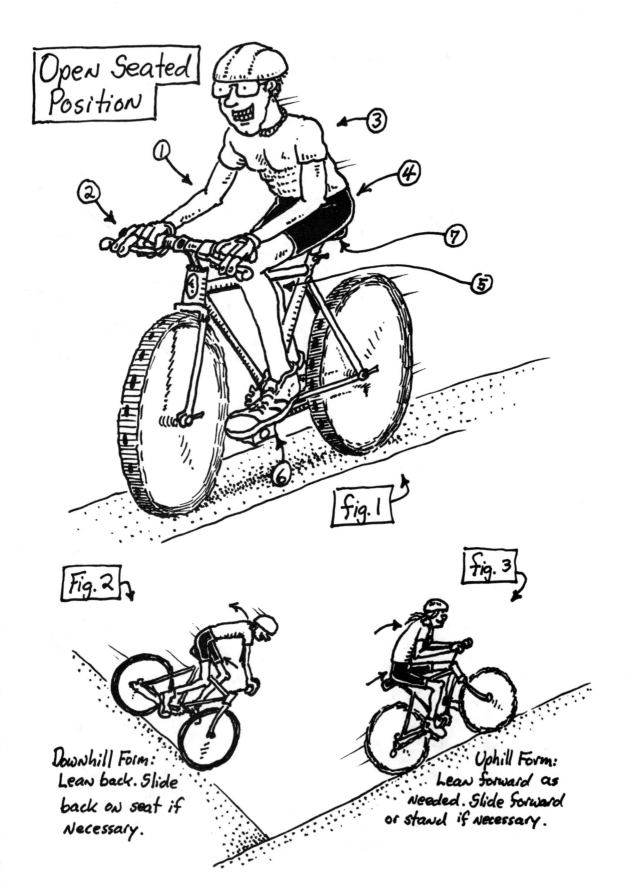

Open Seated Position

fig. 1

Fig. 2

Downhill Form:
Lean back. Slide
back on seat if
necessary.

fig. 3

Uphill Form:
Lean forward as
needed. Slide forward
or stand if necessary.

Your average mtn. biker will spend about 60% of his/her riding time in the Open Seated Position. "Open" means relaxed, comfortable and anatomically spread out. "Closed" (see below) means anatomically compacted and semi-rigid, usually for aerodynamic reasons. In the open seated position the rider is in a neutral muscular attitude above the waist, absorbing shock, leaning, steering and working the brakes. From this position the rider can tuck for maximum speed or stand for greater power & control instantly. This position lies exactly center on the action/non-action continuum.

Fig.1 ① Elbows relaxed, greater than a 90° angle, absorbing shock. ② Hands cradling grips firmly, virtually no weight on bars. ③ Back bowed slightly to absorb shock. ④ Weight distributed between seat and pedals, almost Never fully on seat [see "Stance"] ⑤ Knees flexed, never locked! [See "Crash Protocol"] ⑥ Feet slightly pigeontoed, weight centered on ball of foot. ⑦ Focus of "Cone of Movement" centered on seat. [See "Cone of Movement".]

fig.4 Closed Seated Position [a.k.a. "Tuck"]

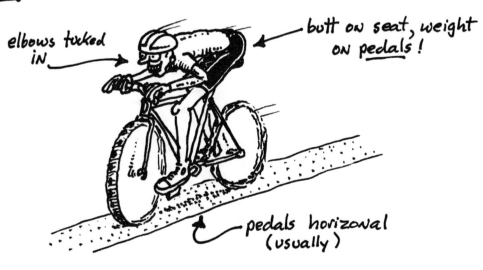

elbows tucked in

butt on seat, weight on pedals!

pedals horizonal (usually)

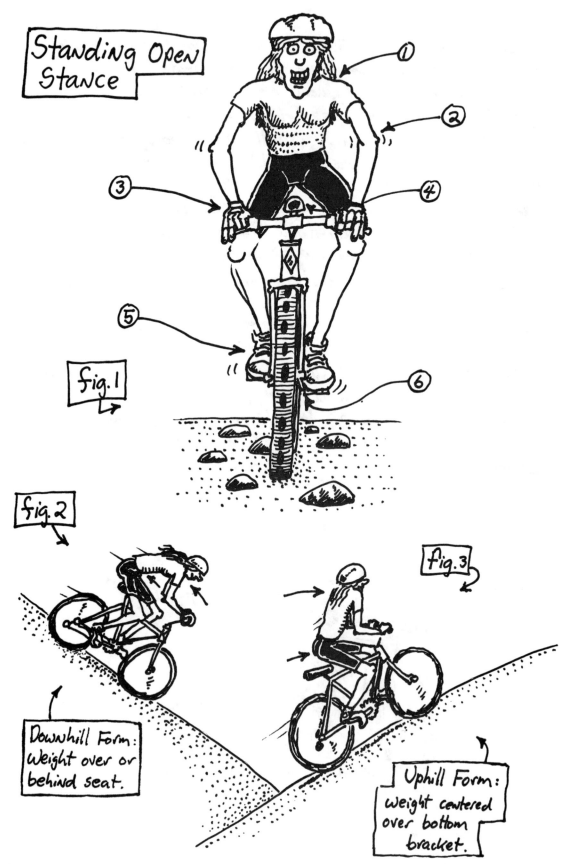

Standing Open Stance

fig.1

fig.2

fig.3

Downhill Form: Weight over or behind seat.

Uphill Form: weight centered over bottom bracket.

The Standing Open Stance is the most active & dynamic position on a mtn. bike. The rider is off the seat with his/her weight on the pedals. All muscles are semi-flexed [See "Muscle Terminology"]. The "cone of movement" is huge compared to sitting and the body becomes a giant shock-absorber.

Fig. 1 ① Back semi-bowed to straight. ② Elbows out, absorbing shock, ready to jerk or shove [See "Armed and Dangerous".] ③ Hands gripping firmly, working with feet for extra power [See pg. 30] ④ Butt off seat, centered over seatpost. ⑤ Feet slightly pigeontoed, 99% of weight on feet. ⑥ Cone of movement focused on bottom bracket.

fig.4 Standing Closed Stance - This is a standing demi-tuck used mainly for high speed descents over rough or loose surfaces.

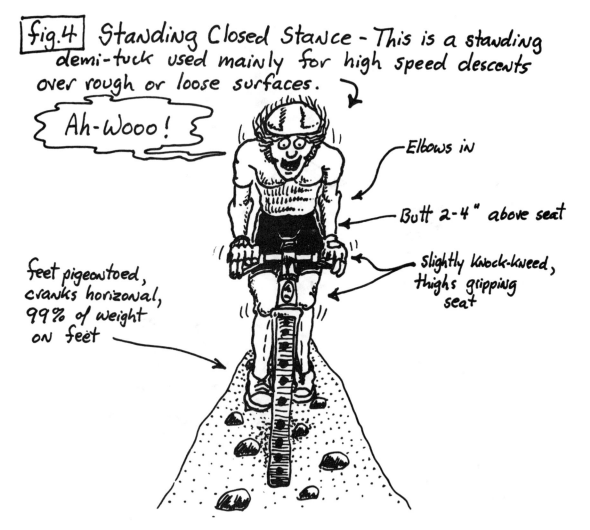

Ah-Wooo!

Elbows in

Butt 2-4" above seat

slightly knock-kneed, thighs gripping seat

feet pigeontoed, cranks horizonal, 99% of weight on feet

Cone of Movement — The amount of lean a rider can exert on his/her bike is determined by the focus of his/her stance: in a seated position, the cone of movement is focused on the seat [fig 1] and is relatively small. The greater the obstacle, the larger the cone of movement must be to surmount it. [See fig. 2, opposite.]

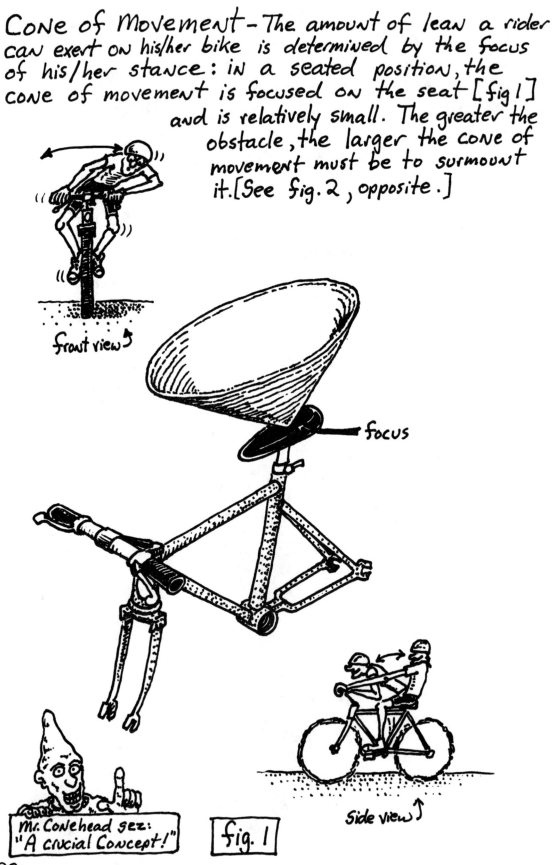

front view ↰

focus

Mr. Conehead sez:
"A crucial Concept!"

fig. 1

side view ↰

From a standing position the cone of movement is huge compared to sitting. This gives the rider an exponentially greater number of options in terms of leans, weight shifts and control.

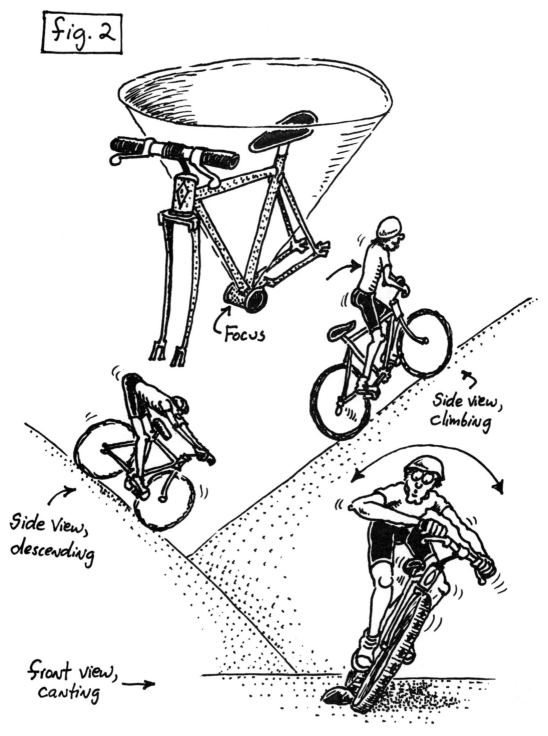

fig. 2

Focus

Side view, climbing

Side view, descending

Front view, canting

Armed And Dangerous...
(Basic Arm Theory)

Armed and Dangerous

Arms are for steering, right? Functionally speaking, actual steering is merely a part-time job. The real work arms perform is suspension and balance. Learning the optimal combinations of arm stiffness and flexion is the key to good trail technique...

Bad Arm Technique I: arms locked, handlebars weighted

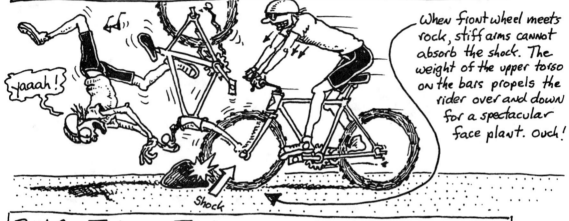

When front wheel meets rock, stiff arms cannot absorb the shock. The weight of the upper torso on the bars propels the rider over and down for a spectacular face plant. ouch!

Bad Arm Technique II: loose arms, handlebars unweighted

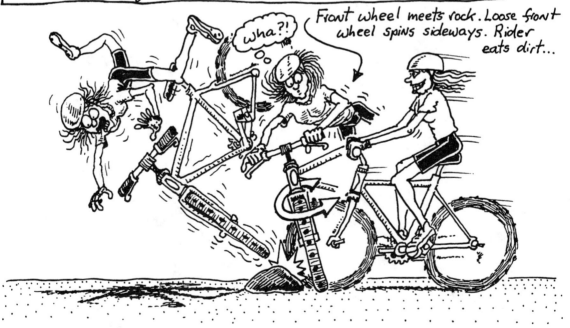

Front wheel meets rock. Loose front wheel spins sideways. Rider eats dirt...

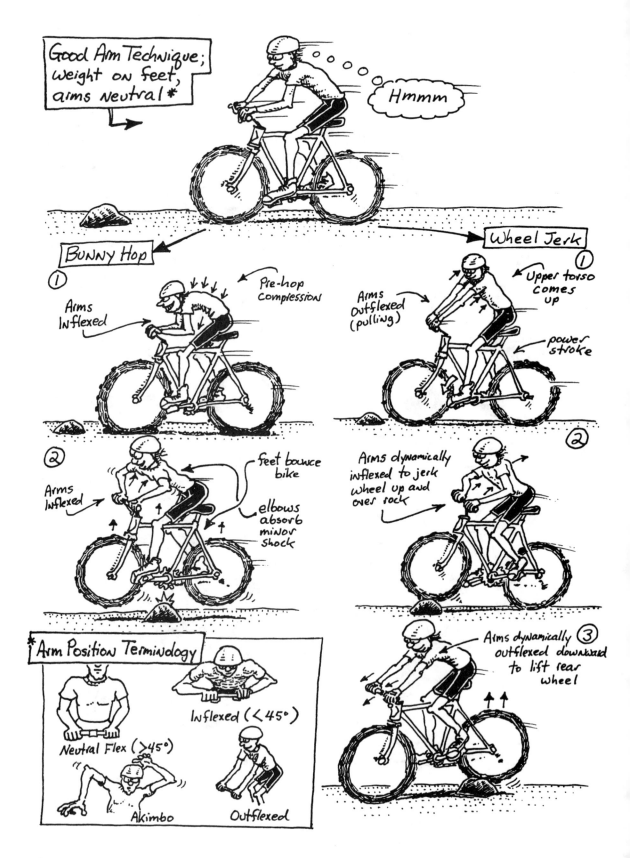

All About Steering... The creative mtn. biker has lots of options when it comes to changing direction on his/her bike...

① "Normal Steering" - This is simply turning the handlebars in combination with a slight inside lean at low to medium speeds. The result is a wide rounded semi-circular turn.

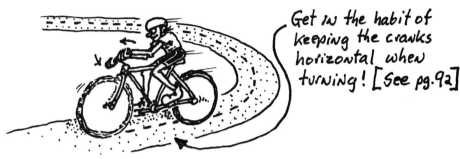

Get in the habit of keeping the cranks horizontal when turning! [See pg. 92]

② Banked Steering - A more dynamic technique utilizing a pronounced inside lean in combination with a slight turn of the bars. You can micro-adjust the turn diameter within the turn by arm & leg swings. Banking is best at moderate to high speeds.

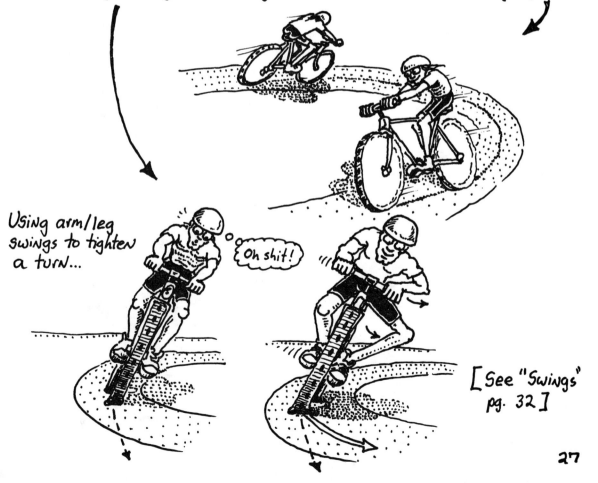

Using arm/leg swings to tighten a turn...

Oh shit!

[See "Swings" pg. 32]

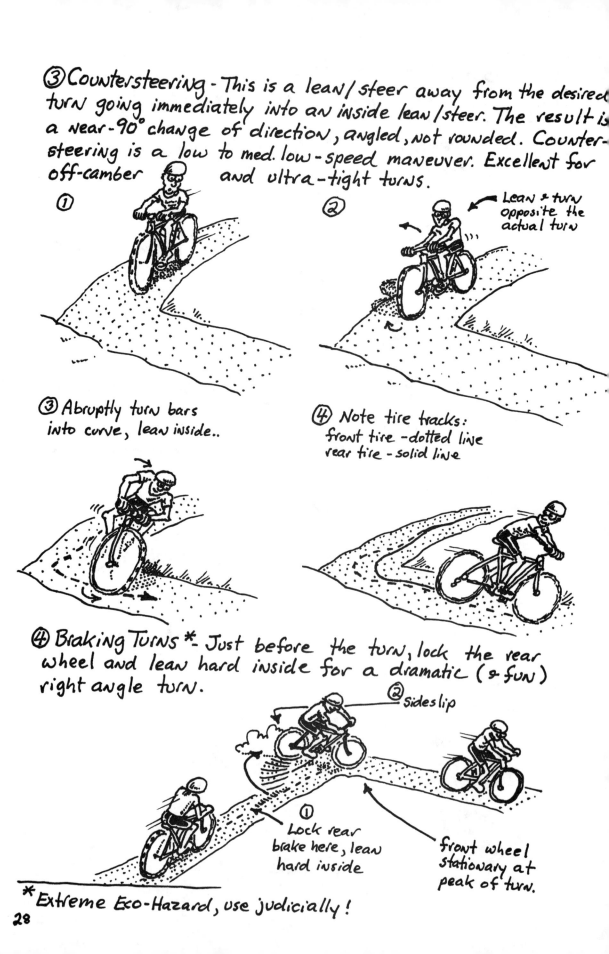

③ **Countersteering** - This is a lean/steer away from the desired turn going immediately into an inside lean/steer. The result is a near-90° change of direction, angled, not rounded. Countersteering is a low to med. low-speed maneuver. Excellent for off-camber and ultra-tight turns.

① ②

Lean & turn opposite the actual turn

③ Abruptly turn bars into curve, lean inside..

④ Note tire tracks:
front tire -dotted line
rear tire - solid line

④ **Braking Turns *** - Just before the turn, lock the rear wheel and lean hard inside for a dramatic (& fun) right angle turn.

② sideslip

① Lock rear brake here, lean hard inside

front wheel stationary at peak of turn.

* Extreme Eco-Hazard, use judicially!

28

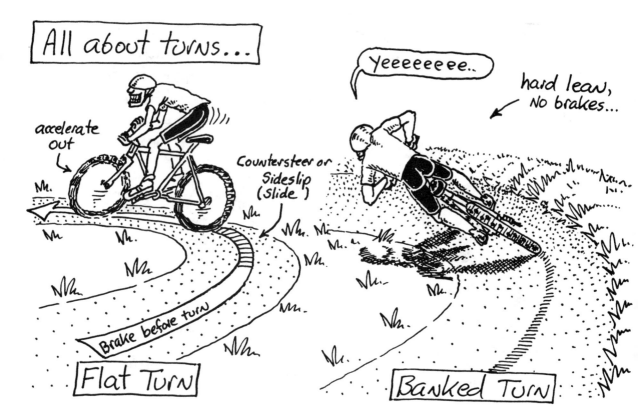

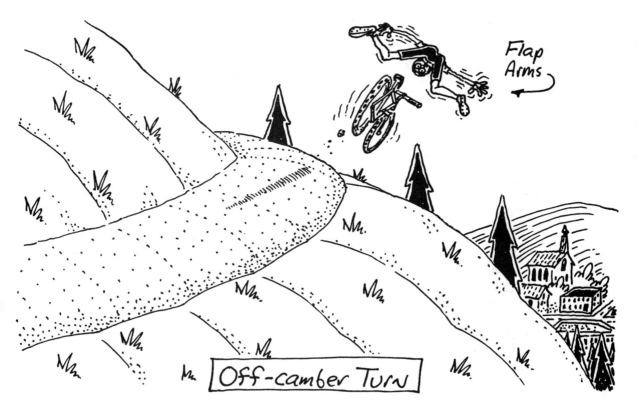

Arm-assisted Power Strokes

In normal pedalling a rider cannot exert more force on the pedals than he/she weighs, usually only a fraction thereof. But a strong pull on the handlebars in conjunction with hard pedal strokes allows the rider to exert greater-than-body weight on the cranks. [figs. 1 & 2]

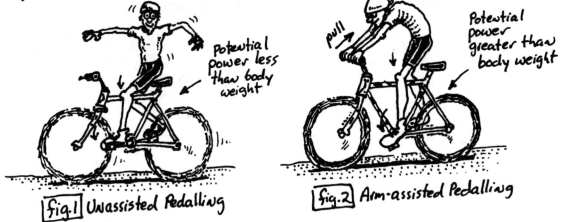

Potential power less than body weight

fig.1 Unassisted Pedalling

pull

Potential power greater than body weight

fig.2 Arm-assisted Pedalling

By using an arm-pull in opposition to the downward push on the pedals you add tremendous power by increasing your leverage on the powertrain. Pulling on the right grip against a right pedal stroke is a "same side assist" and gives you almost maximum torque..

Note: Arm-pull assists are almost always done from a standing position.

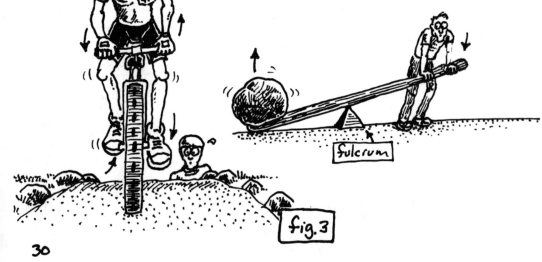

gasp!

fulcrum

fig.3

To achieve absolute maximum power and torque, pull hard on the grip opposite the pedal stroke. This increases the length of your body lever. Using "opposed arm assists also causes the bike to cant (see below) [See pp 44-45]

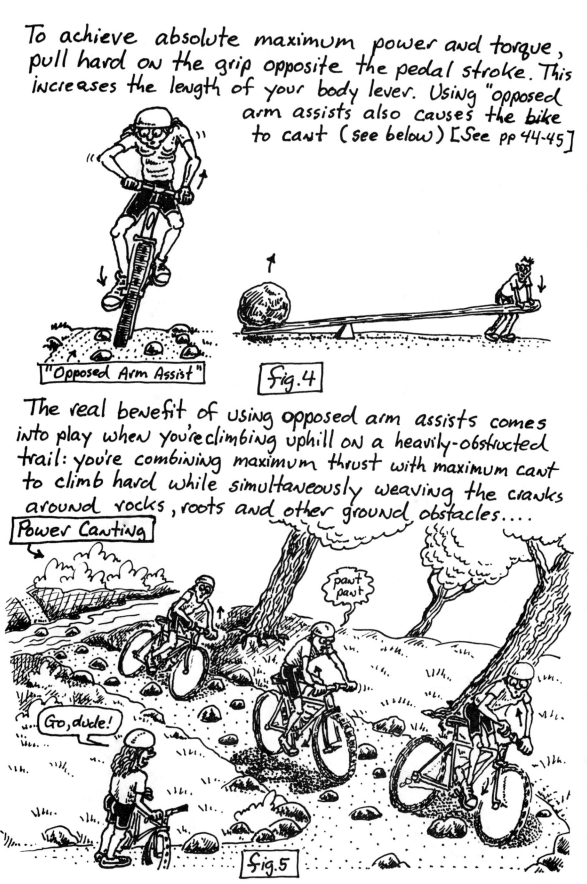

"Opposed Arm Assist"

fig. 4

The real benefit of using opposed arm assists comes into play when you're climbing uphill on a heavily-obstructed trail: you're combining maximum thrust with maximum cant to climb hard while simultaneously weaving the cranks around rocks, roots and other ground obstacles....

Power Canting

pant pant

Go, dude!

fig. 5

Swings Use arm and leg "swings" when banking to micro-adjust your bike's attitude in the turn...

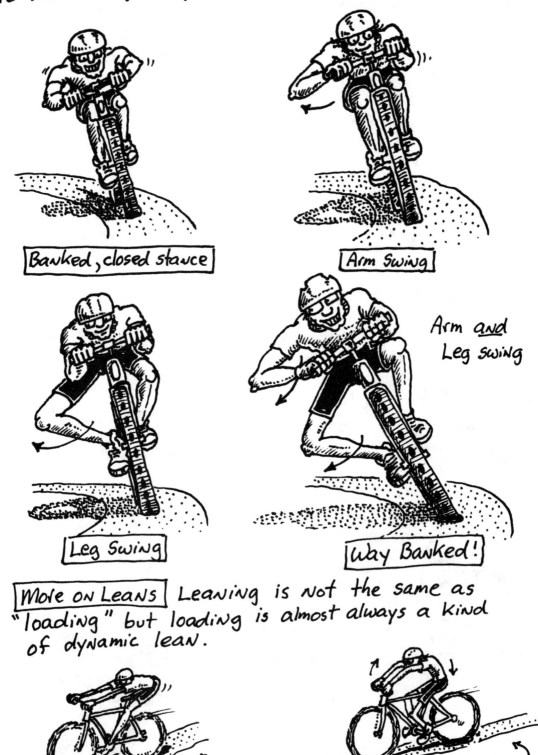

Banked, closed stance

Arm Swing

Leg Swing

Arm and Leg swing

Way Banked!

More on Leans Leaning is not the same as "loading" but loading is almost always a kind of dynamic lean.

Rear Leaning

Rear wheel Loading

Vertical Loading/Unloading The next diagrams show several methods of loading and unloading one or both wheels to aid in crossing or hopping a variety of low obstacles. **Front Wheel Micro-hop** This is dynamic weighting of the front wheel to pop it suddenly an inch or so off the ground. Also a lead-in to the Wheelie Hop.

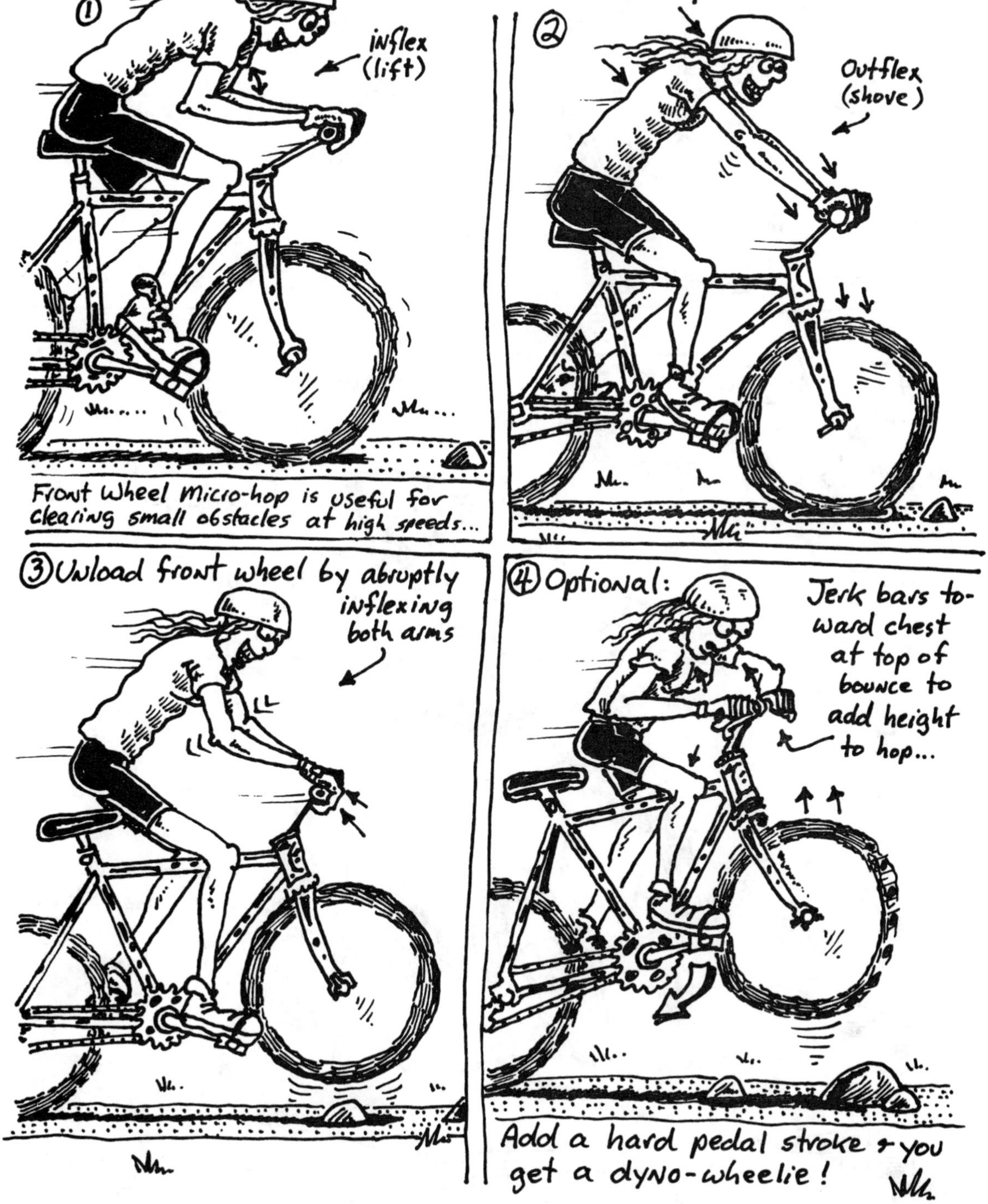

① inflex (lift)

Front wheel micro-hop is useful for clearing small obstacles at high speeds...

② Outflex (shove)

③ Unload front wheel by abruptly inflexing both arms

④ Optional: Jerk bars toward chest at top of bounce to add height to hop...

Add a hard pedal stroke & you get a dyno-wheelie!

33

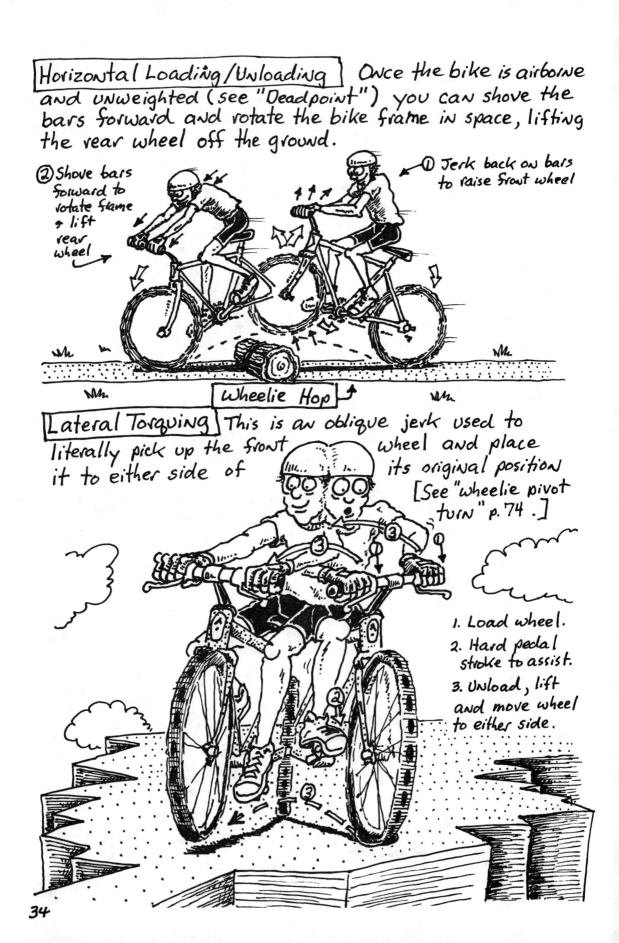

Horizontal Loading/Unloading Once the bike is airborne and unweighted (see "Deadpoint") you can shove the bars forward and rotate the bike frame in space, lifting the rear wheel off the ground.

② Shove bars forward to rotate frame & lift rear wheel

① Jerk back on bars to raise front wheel

Wheelie Hop

Lateral Torquing This is an oblique jerk used to literally pick up the front wheel and place it to either side of its original position [See "wheelie pivot turn" p.74.]

1. Load wheel.
2. Hard pedal stroke to assist.
3. Unload, lift and move wheel to either side.

34

Basic Handlebar Torque Concept

By pushing and pulling on opposite grips you can rotate the frame around the short axis of the bike. Torquing the bars is mainly used in "power canting" but from a "Deadpoint" you can use sudden bar-torque to twitch the bike upright after a near knockdown (fig.2).

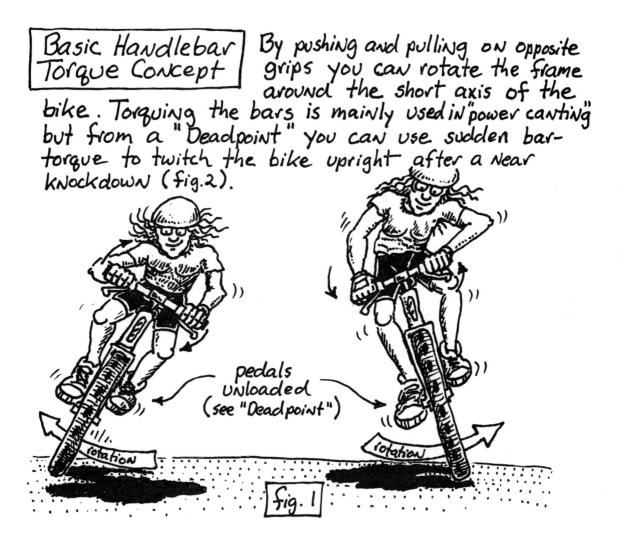

pedals
unloaded
(see "Deadpoint")

rotation

rotation

fig. 1

Leg / Powertrain Theory

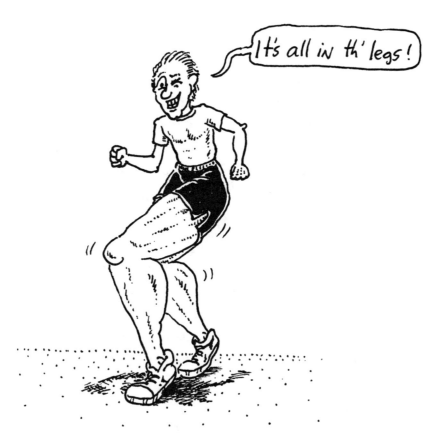

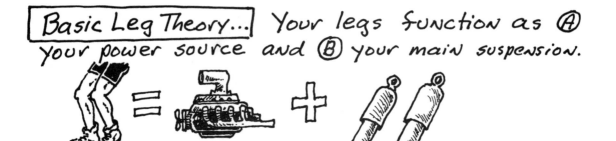

Basic Leg Theory...
Your legs function as Ⓐ your power source and Ⓑ your main suspension.

The trick is to train your legs to perform both functions simultaneously all the time. On trail, the advanced mtn. biker never really puts all his/her weight on the seat even when "fully" seated. By keeping your legs semi-flexed full-time your weight is always focused on the pedals and the seat becomes largely superfluous except as a reference point. If you're riding seated with the right amount of leg flexion, you will be able to move from the seat to a semi-crouched upright position (the standard trail position) in an easy, fluid motion.

engine
transmission
drive shaft
differential

  The secret of excellent leg technique is gear shifting so as to maintain a fairly constant r.p.m. on the pedals combined with a constant and appropriate amount of pressure on the pedals [see "Shift Discipline"]. For example, if you're climbing a super-steep pitch and you accidentally drop three gears on the downshift you will loose traction, balance & rhythm (at best!). If you're a dude, you might resultingly find yourself singing soprano with the Vienna Boys' Choir. Obviously, you want to learn to avoid shifting too low/too far/too soon. Fluidity and finesse are what count in on-trail shifting, not brute strength! Here's a highly educational leg technique experiment you can try... (heh heh)... take your seat off, hide it in the bushes and ride about an hour on your favorite trail. If your legs are fully blown after about 15 minutes you are definately a "Seat Junkie!" Put your seat back on and concentrate on riding with only half your weight on the seat. You should find this much less exhausting than riding seatless, as well as being smoother obstaclewise. You have just demonstrated to your legs the correct amount of seated leg-flexion for on-trail use. The next trick to teach your legs is the "micro-rest." This is a technique whereby each leg gets a teeny little nap on the backside of each crank revolution (see below).

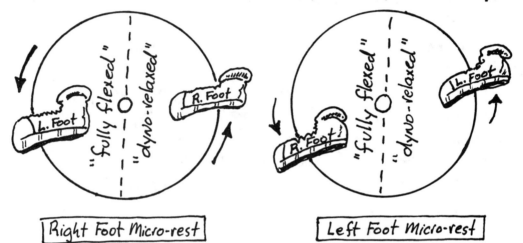

Right Foot Micro-rest   Left Foot Micro-rest

This may seem insignificant at first but on a half-mile plus uphill hump it really works if done right! If you're using the power stroke to lift the "resting leg" you are doing it wrong. Ideally you want to suddenly relax the resting leg and do the lifting with your abdominal muscles. A micro-rest works by allowing arteries and veins in a hard-working muscle group to expand between contractions to allow additional inflow of oxygen and outflow of CO_2 and lactic acid. Keep in mind that micro-resting is a specialized technique to be used occasionally under duress. Good pedalling technique requires both legs to be working: one leg pushing down, the other leg lifting up ⟶

Note: Micro-resting transforms anaerobic muscle activity into aerobic muscle activity!

"Fully Flexed" "semi-flexed"

toe clips a must!

"Normal Pedalling Technique"

39

The ultimate test for good leg technique is steep "pitch climbing." While humping up a multi-mile fire-road upgrade is a test of mere endurance and shifting strategy, climbing a short, steep, irregularly-surfaced uphill section of trail requires the rider to dynamically combine maximum power, maximum shock absorption, superior shifting and advanced lean techniques _perfectly_ to reach the top still on the pedals.

There are two divergent philosophies on optimal body position for serious climbing situations:
① Climbing Seated School - these guys say to hunker down on the seat and pedal furiously to top any hill.
② Climbing Standing School - these guys insist that climbing upright is the one true way to conquer all steep uphill stretches. Both techniques work pretty well and the rider who can master both styles will effectively double his/her options for approaching all climbing situations. Both styles have their drawbacks as well as strengths...

Climbing Seated Arguably the best routine climbing technique, especially on loose surfaces, because your body position is centered and stays very stable, insuring excellent traction...

Eeeyow!

pant... gasp... pant...

However, if the up-grade is inconsistent and/or bumpy, and/or if you're using too low a gear, you will probably burn out your legs long before you reach the top. Climbing standing is much less exhausting than climbing seated in too low a gear!!

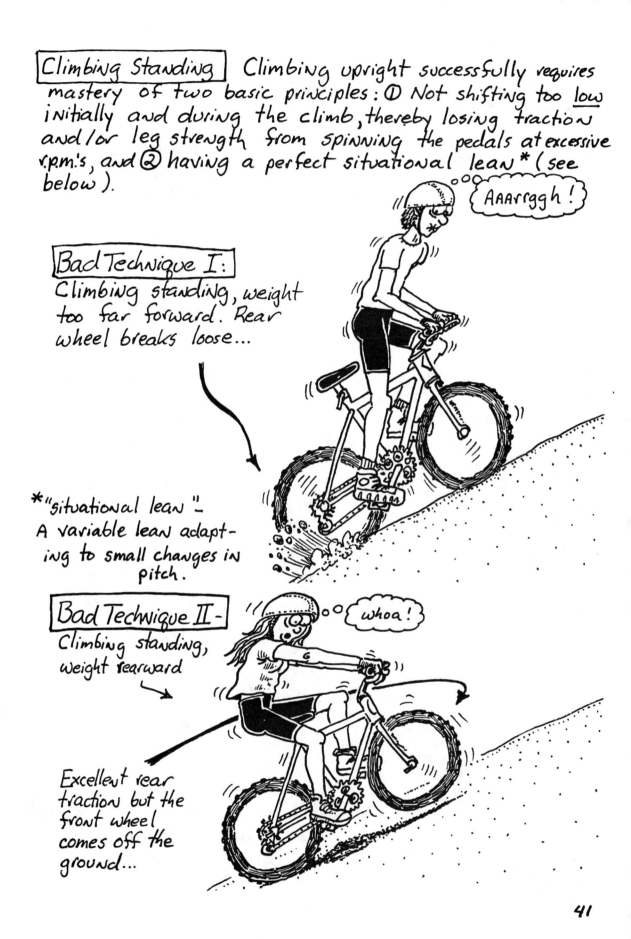

Climbing Standing   Climbing upright successfully requires mastery of two basic principles: ① Not shifting too low initially and during the climb, thereby losing traction and/or leg strength from spinning the pedals at excessive r.p.m.'s, and ② having a perfect situational lean* (see below).

Aaarrggh!

Bad Technique I:
Climbing standing, weight too far forward. Rear wheel breaks loose...

*"situational lean"—
A variable lean adapting to small changes in pitch.

Bad Technique II—
Climbing standing, weight rearward

whoa!

Excellent rear traction but the front wheel comes off the ground...

You get a lot more power from climbing standing but most of your mental energy is wasted on maintaining perfectly centered weight distribution. Also, energetic standing pedaling makes the bike unstable and more likely to lose traction on loose surfaces...

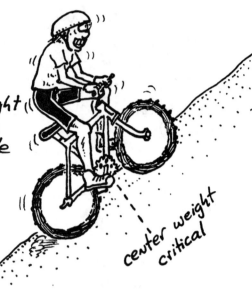

center weight critical

Where climbing standing really excels is on very steep & uneven trials grades. Attempting such a grade seated requires the rider to start & stay in too low a gear or to shift up & down one gear to maintain constant pedal r.p.m. By standing and staying in a relatively higher gear without shifting, your pedal cadence will vary some but overall smoothness will be far superior to climbing seated. Standing, you always have much more available power!

Also, climbing standing on a real bumpy upgrade saves lots of wear and tear on one's naughty parts !!!

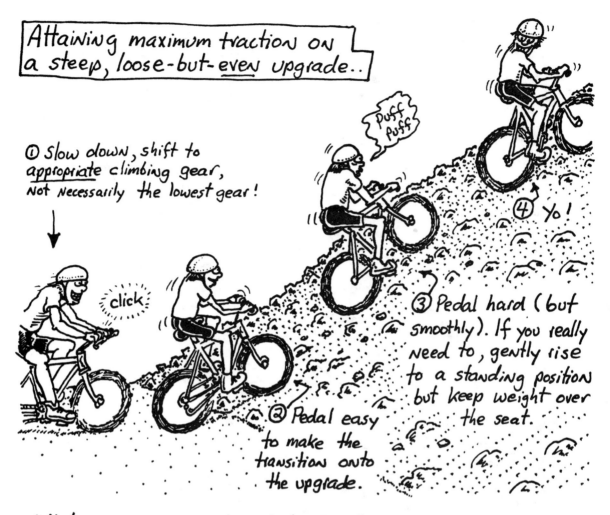

Attaining maximum traction on a steep, loose-but-_even_ upgrade..

① Slow down, shift to appropriate climbing gear, not necessarily the lowest gear!

click

② Pedal easy to make the transition onto the upgrade.

Puff Puff

④ Yo!

③ Pedal hard (but smoothly). If you really need to, gently rise to a standing position but keep weight over the seat.

While you always want to be fluid when moving from seated to standing and back, normally on a hard upgrade you will only be moving from seated to standing because moving from standing to sitting causes a dramatic net loss of power. Once you stand on a steep pitch, remain standing and avoid shifting at all!

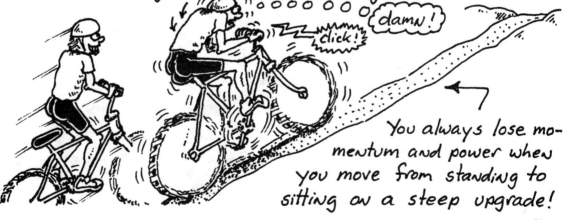

o o o o o o o o

click!

damn!

You always lose momentum and power when you move from standing to sitting on a steep upgrade!

Advanced Leg Techniques: Ratcheting and Canting...

At some point in your mtn. biking career you're sure to encounter a stretch of trail so festooned with rocks & roots that normal pedalling is impossible because your pedals, cranks, chainwheel and derailleur are hanging up...

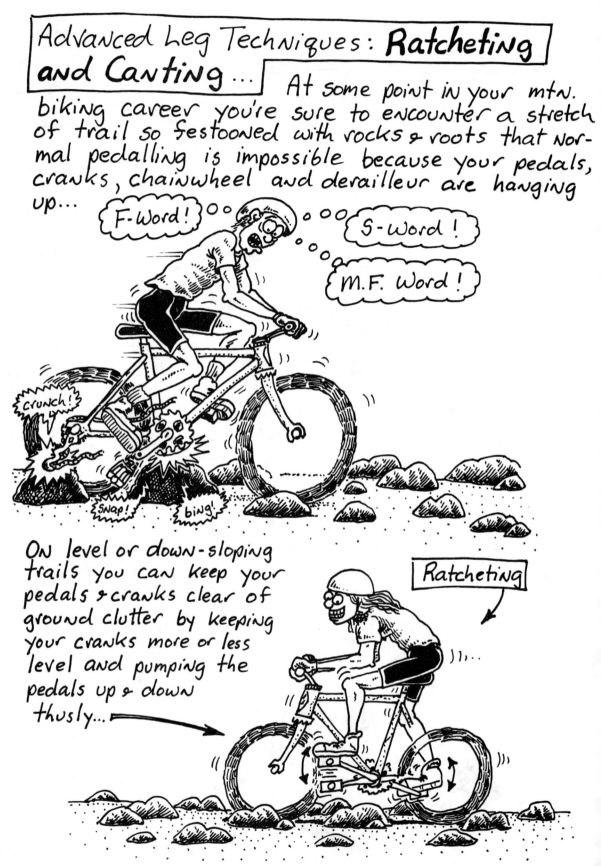

On level or down-sloping trails you can keep your pedals & cranks clear of ground clutter by keeping your cranks more or less level and pumping the pedals up & down thusly...

On upgrades where ratcheting is impossible you can "cant" the bike on the down stroke of the pedal and gain 2" of additional ground clearance for pedals & up to 1" for the chainwheel and derailleur.

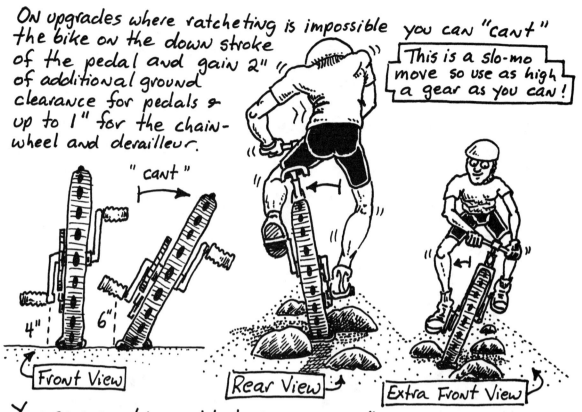

"This is a slo-mo move so use as high a gear as you can!"

"cant"

4" 6"

Front View

Rear View

Extra Front View

You can combine ratchet strokes and "cant" moves to deal with the gnarliest terrain imaginable...

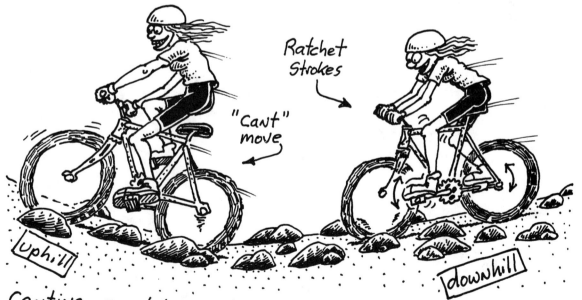

Ratchet Strokes

"Cant" move

uphill

downhill

Canting your bike is also a good way to fit your handlebars thru trees spaced closer together than handlebar width...

Using Legs & Arms To Load/Unload The Wheels...

By suddenly shifting your weight forward and backward you can dynamically affect the behavior of your bike. A hard forward weight shift with a hard downward punch on the handlebars loads (compresses) the front wheel for a front wheel hop and, when airborne, lifts the rear wheel (fig.1).

Front Wheel Loading On the Ground..

Front Wheel Loading In the Air...

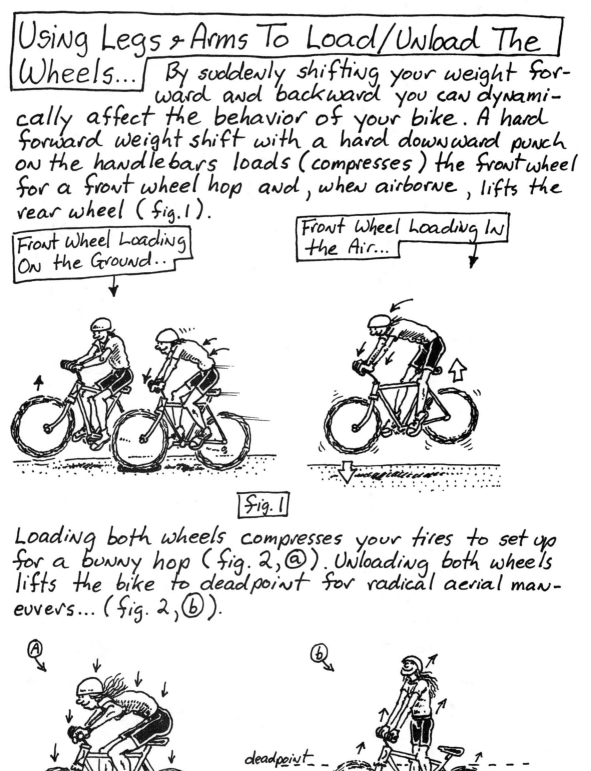

Fig. 1

Loading both wheels compresses your tires to set up for a bunny hop (fig. 2,ⓐ). Unloading both wheels lifts the bike to deadpoint for radical aerial maneuvers... (fig. 2,ⓑ).

ⓐ

ⓑ

deadpoint

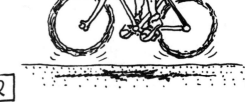

fig.2

46

Loading the rear wheel enhances a wheelie or, when airborne, raises the front wheel for a good landing attitude...

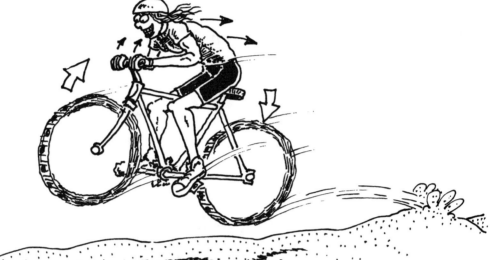

You can also do a rear wheel hop (a relatively useless bike trick) by jabbing your butt toward the headset and lunging forward. If you do this at low speed combined with a locked front wheel you can actually do a front wheel pivot turn (another relatively useless bike trick compared to other turning options).

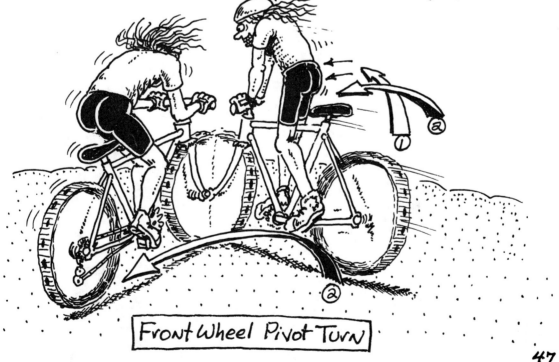

Front Wheel Pivot Turn

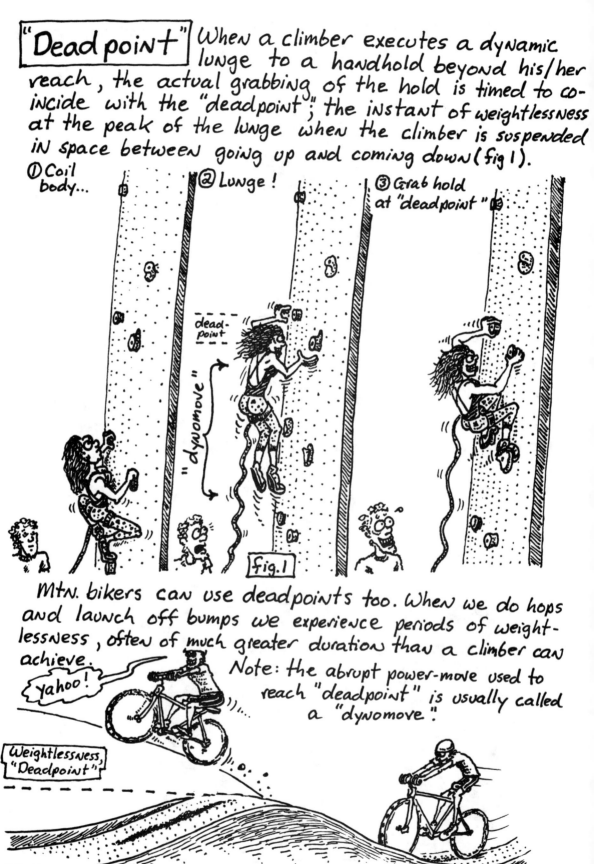

"Deadpoint" When a climber executes a dynamic lunge to a handhold beyond his/her reach, the actual grabbing of the hold is timed to co-incide with the "deadpoint"; the instant of weightlessness at the peak of the lunge when the climber is suspended in space between going up and coming down (fig 1).

① Coil body...

② Lunge!

③ Grab hold at "deadpoint"

deadpoint

"dynomove"

fig. 1

Mtn. bikers can use deadpoints too. When we do hops and launch off bumps we experience periods of weight-lessness, often of much greater duration than a climber can achieve.

yahoo!

Note: the abrupt power-move used to reach "deadpoint" is usually called a "dynomove."

Weightlessness, "Deadpoint"

The deadpoint is a key concept in the mastery of the bunny hop, wheelie hop and most aerial maneuvers...

③ Jerk bike higher off ground! (Dynamic Recoil)

② Lunge (unload wheels)

① Dynamic coil (load wheels)

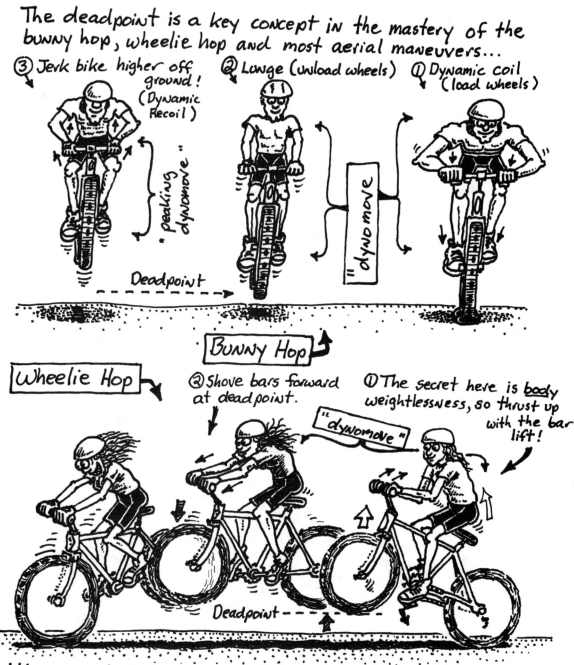

"peaking dynomove"

Deadpoint

"dyno move"

Wheelie Hop

Bunny Hop

② Shove bars forward at deadpoint.

① The secret here is **body** weightlessness, so thrust up with the bar lift!

"dynomove"

Deadpoint

It's easier to peak a move at "deadpoint" because it takes far more energy to set in motion an object weighing several hundred pounds (curb weight of you plus your bike) than it does to set in motion an object weighing a few ounces (you & your bike at "deadpoint"). You can learn "deadpointing" by pogoing on your bike until you're achieving distinct points of weightlessness at the top of each bounce. Now it's just a matter of adding more power to your lunge ("dynomove").

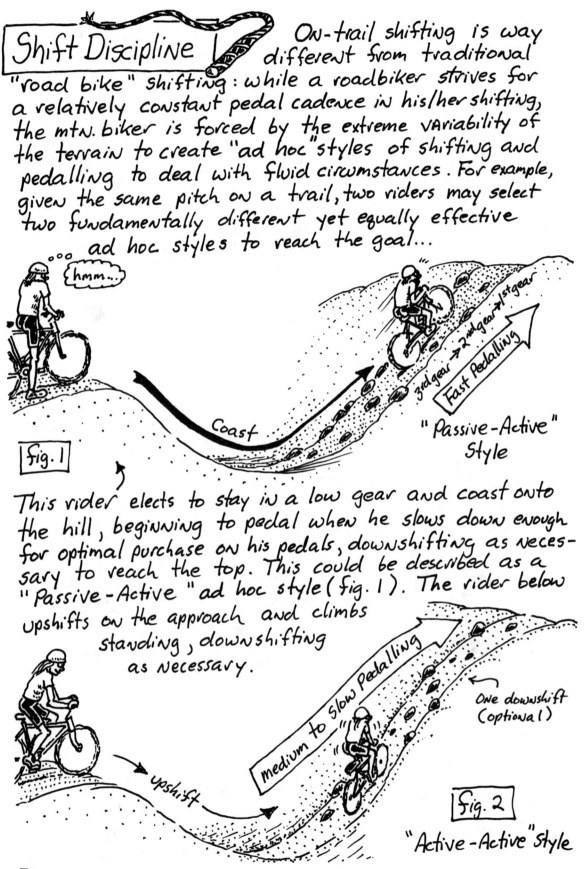

Shift Discipline

On-trail shifting is way different from traditional "road bike" shifting: while a roadbiker strives for a relatively constant pedal cadence in his/her shifting, the mtn. biker is forced by the extreme variability of the terrain to create "ad hoc" styles of shifting and pedalling to deal with fluid circumstances. For example, given the same pitch on a trail, two riders may select two fundamentally different yet equally effective ad hoc styles to reach the goal...

hmm...

Coast

3rd gear → 2nd gear → 1st gear

Fast Pedalling

fig. 1

"Passive-Active" Style

This rider elects to stay in a low gear and coast onto the hill, beginning to pedal when he slows down enough for optimal purchase on his pedals, downshifting as necessary to reach the top. This could be described as a "Passive-Active" ad hoc style (fig. 1). The rider below upshifts on the approach and climbs standing, downshifting as necessary.

upshift

medium to slow Pedalling

One downshift (optional)

fig. 2

"Active-Active" Style

This could be described as an "Active-Active" approach: the rider pedals and shifts all the way through while the "Passive-Active" rider does his shifting and pedalling in a burst. The best style is the style that suits <u>you</u> <u>and your particular circumstances.</u>

Rules of Good Shift Discipline :

· <u>Rule #1</u> - There are no rules, only options !

"<u>Shift Option</u>"#2 - Use your gears, that's what they're there for.

<u>Shift Option</u>#3 - If you stay on the middle chainwheel and middle gears, you can reduce chain-wear and virtually eliminate "chain suck."

<u>Shift Option</u> #4 - Maintain a smooth cadence and conserve energy by riding seated and going through the gears (moderate up-grades or severe up-grades with loose surfaces)

<u>Shift Option</u> #5 Maintain smoothness & fluidity while attaining maximum climbing torque by standing on the pedals on the highest gear you can tolerate, and avoiding/minimizing down-shifts (ultra-steep bumpy upgrade, packed surface).

<u>Shift Option</u> #6 - Save the granny gear for the very top of a hill. Move from seated to standing position if necessary.

<u>Shift Option</u> #7 - When anticipating a standing climb, decide on the optimal gear for the grade and shift to the next <u>highest</u> gear ! This compensates for a psychological anomalie wherein the gear the rider pre-selects for a standing climb is almost always one gear too low.

<u>Shift Option</u> #8 - Use the granny gear minimally on hard climbs ! Pedalling way too fast is ultimately far more exhausting than pedalling hard and slow.

<u>Shift Option</u> #9 - If you're bouncing over bumpy terrain at moderate to high speeds, shift to a higher than necessary gear to maintain tension on your chain (see "chain suck") <u>Shift Option</u> #10 Avoid using the front shifter to downshift under hard standing-pedalling circumstances! (see "Pedalling Air", following pages).

Chainwheel Detail

Big Chainring
a.k.a. "tree crampon"
a.k.a. "road gear"

Middle Chainring
a.k.a. "Cruising gear"
a.k.a. "DRIVE"

Small Chainring
a.k.a. "Front Granny Gear"
a.k.a. "Low"

Freewheel Detail

low

High

"Low-low or granny gear"

6th 5th 4th 3rd 2nd 1st

PLEASE NOTE: The author refers to gears just like manual-shift automotive gears: 1st gear = "low" (large gear on freewheel / small gear on chainwheel), 6th gear = "high" (small gear on freewheel / large gear on chainwheel). Shifting from a high gear to a lower gear is a "downshift," from a low gear to a high gear is an "upshift."

Consequences of Poor Shift Discipline:

"Leg Burn"- What happens when your legs get oxygen starved and lactic acid overdosed from pedalling either too fast in a too-low gear or too hard in a too-high gear. In both cases the muscles of the leg are over-contracted to the extent that inflow of O_2 and outflow of CO_2 & lactic acid are restricted. The rider must learn to chose the optimal gear(s) for any situation and modify his/her pedalling technique to build "micro-rests" into the pedal strokes.

Whaaa?

52

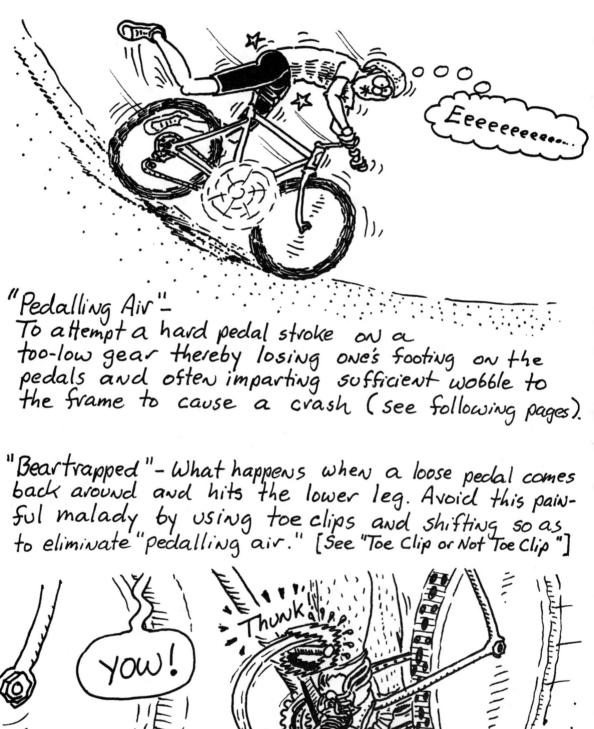

"Pedalling Air"-
To attempt a hard pedal stroke on a too-low gear thereby losing one's footing on the pedals and often imparting sufficient wobble to the frame to cause a crash (see following pages).

"Beartrapped" - What happens when a loose pedal comes back around and hits the lower leg. Avoid this painful malady by using toe clips and shifting so as to eliminate "pedalling air." [See "Toe Clip or Not Toe Clip"]

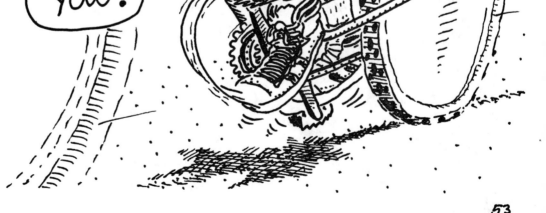

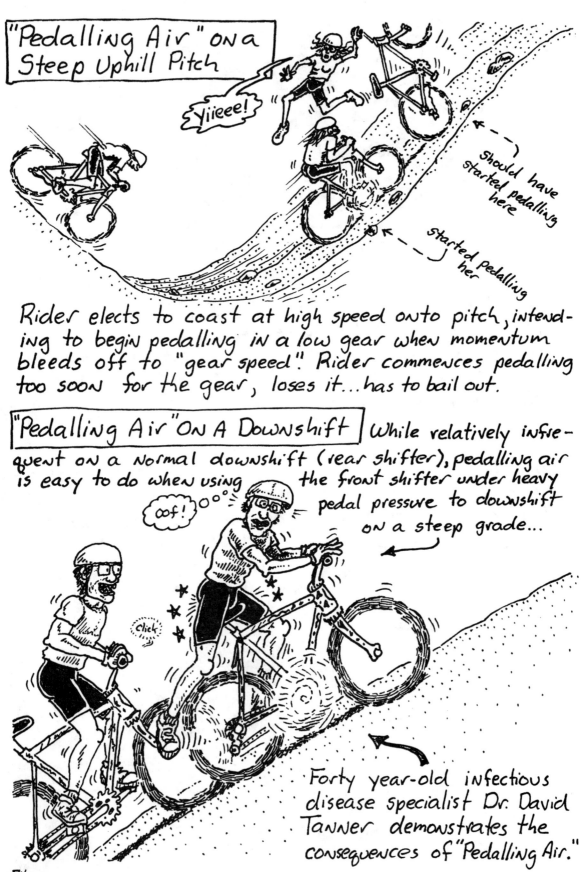

"Pedalling Air" on a Steep Uphill Pitch

Yiieee!

Should have started pedalling here

started pedalling her

Rider elects to coast at high speed onto pitch, intending to begin pedalling in a low gear when momentum bleeds off to "gear speed". Rider commences pedalling too soon for the gear, loses it...has to bail out.

"Pedalling Air" on a Downshift While relatively infrequent on a normal downshift (rear shifter), pedalling air is easy to do when using the front shifter under heavy pedal pressure to downshift on a steep grade...

oof! oooo

click

Forty year-old infectious disease specialist Dr. David Tanner demonstrates the consequences of "Pedalling Air."

Caterpillaring While coasting is perfectly acceptable under most conditions, failure to pre-select the correct gear for when you resume pedalling can result in cluster downshifting and/or furious pedalling to compensate for the bad selection. Viewed from a distance, the rider appears to be creeping down the trail like an inch-worm caterpillar, fast-slow, fast slow, etc.

Cadence: low, then high speed.

Cadence: zero

downshift
downshift
downshift

Coasting

Cluster shifting

Above is a great example of bad anticipation: the rider tries to take the hill too fast in a too-high gear. He/she bleeds off too much speed before resuming pedalling. The gear is too high, so the rider downshifts in search of a do-able gear and the delay causes him/her to lose it altogether. A better approach would be to skip the coasting part and run smoothly down through the gears with a much steadier pedalling cadence.

Chain Suck

Shit!

Screech

Almost always caused by going fast on bumps in too low a gear. If you generally keep to the higher gears on bumps there will be more tension on the chain making it much less likely to flop between the chainstay and the tire.

Learning "Anticipation" Good anticipation on the trail is really only a matter of looking ahead, reading the terrain, and planning (in a matter of seconds, usually) the correct sequence of moves necessary to overcome the obstacle(s) ahead. This may sound complicated but, in actual practice, usually isn't. You scan a complex-looking trail section for the most difficult move needed and time everything backwards from there. The most difficult move on a given stretch of trail is a "peak move". All other necessary body movements are built around this move in a fluid move sequence.

Peak Move

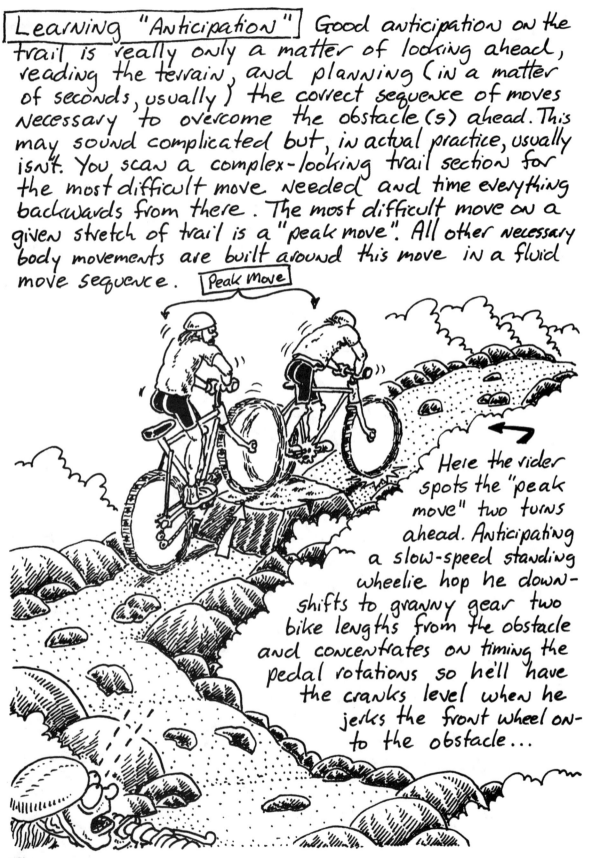

Here the rider spots the "peak move" two turns ahead. Anticipating a slow-speed standing wheelie hop he downshifts to granny gear two bike lengths from the obstacle and concentrates on timing the pedal rotations so he'll have the cranks level when he jerks the front wheel onto the obstacle...

Watch a really good rider negotiate a gnarly stretch of "trials" trail. The main thing you'll notice is how simple the rider makes it look. Herein lies the essence of mastering the hard stuff: <u>simplicity</u> and <u>Negotiation</u>. The advanced rider "reads" the future-trail and conforms body and bike to the obstacle, flowing over it with the absolute minimum of moves and exertion. Watch a novice try to <u>force</u> the same stretch of trail: he/she invariably tries to beat the trail into submission with flailing body-moves and incredible exertion only to lose it from sheer exhaustion and/or loss of traction from overpowering the bike. Don't try to force the trail, fit yourself through it!

Here's where anticipation comes in. On a tricky stretch of trail your average novice quickly falls victim to "porpoising"— instead of driving the bike, the bike drives them! If you're riding down a trail at a decent speed (8-12 mph) and hit a series of obstacles, you will lose control of the bike if you try to react serially to each obstacle! Figuratively speaking, your brain gets further and further behind the bike and you go boom!

| Porpoising |

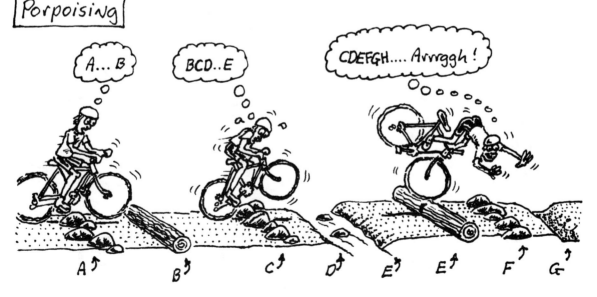

On the other hand, the advanced rider rides focused several moves ahead, constantly pushing the bike toward an ever-receding goal. Reaction to an immediate obstacle is automatic and preconscious ("body knowledge") for the most part. In other words, the advanced rider isn't really reacting to obstacles so much as he/she is following a series of pre-programmed body moves while simultaneously programming the next series of moves.

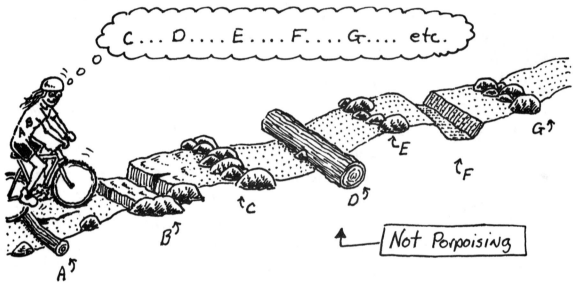

All this may sound complicated but you do it every day... for instance, when you drive a car you're not reacting to the pavement immediately in front of the wheel and thinking "steer... brake... gas... check the speedometer.... steer.... etc" unless you're my mom. A normal driver is just smoothly cruising along subconsciously adapting to the road and probably listening to loud rock and roll while grabbing at his/her boy/girlfriend.

All of which, finally, brings us to "focus." When you're learning to mtn. bike (or drive or ski or kayak, etc) you tend to focus on the next immediate obstacle and screen out everything else. This works ok at first when you're going slow but once you move to higher and higher speeds, bike speed at some point exceeds brain speed, causing you to porpoise and lose control. This selective close-focus I call "micro-focus". Under the right circumstances micro-focus can be useful (see below) but most of the time a rider should use "macro-focus," looking at the whole trail from immediately beneath the bike to the event horizon (maximum sight distance). If you're seeing this way you'll find yourself anticipating, not reacting. Micro-focus is reserved for "peak moves" on particularly challenging "trials" stretches of trail.

Micro-focus

Macro-focus

Event Horizon

Summary: Learning "Anticipation"

① Look at the _whole_ trail ahead of you. [macro-focus]
② Concentrate on the peak move(s). [micro-focus]
③ Practice by repeating difficult trail sections, subtracting all unnecessary rider movement. ["move minimalism"]
④ Strive to cut total exertion on a given pitch to the bare minimum to conserve energy and keep the bike "still". This will greatly enhance your smoothness & fluidity. [energy minimalism]
⑤ Keep your mind at least one bikelength ahead of the bike! (see below)

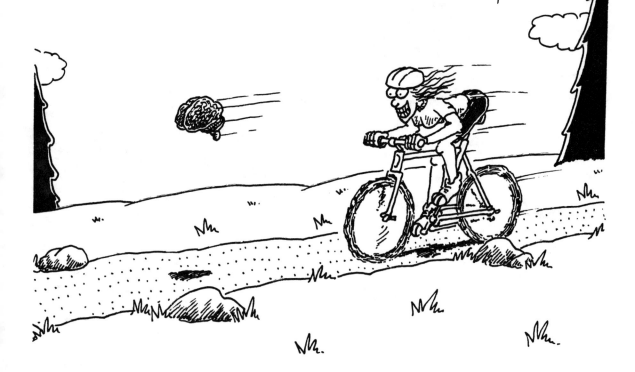

Basic And Advanced Moves

The most challenging part of mountain biking is learning to deal with the huge variety of obstacles we intentionally encounter on trails and elsewhere. Overcoming most any obstacle, fortunately, requires connecting ("chaining") only a few basic moves. It does get pretty complex when you're attempting a long series of obstacles on a typical "fun" "trials trail". However, once you're dealing with a combination of obstacles, the number of potential "obstacle solutions" available to you grows exponentially. Until riding the gnarly stuff becomes instinctual (attainment of "Body knowledge", advanced level), you may want to stop and literally plan out a strategy on trail sections with major obstacle combinations. Study the stretch, formulate your solution (chain of obstacle-solving moves), and try it out...

Wow... creek crossing, deep mud, dodge the rocks, hop the log, can't the boulders... whew!

Obviously the only sane route to "trials trail" mastery is to start out on simple, easy terrain, instinctualize the basic moves and move up the skill ladder incrementally. If you throw yourself at obstacles six notches above your personal skill level, you're going to Ⓐ get hurt and/or Ⓑ get frustrated to the extent that when you

64

<u>are</u> physically & mentally ready for more difficult obstacles you'll have to overcome some psychological obstacles first. Do challenge yourself ontrail but use the "Rule of Fun" ("Am I having fun or is this a psycho-sexual ego crisis?") to avoid unnecessary mental obstacles.

   You probably don't have to look much farther than your front yard for the basic obstacles to practice your basic moves on...

① Down the steps — ("Trail Equivalent" or "T.E." — rocky stairsteps)
② Off the planter & curb — ("T.E." — medium height multi-drop-off)
③ Up & over the curb (T.E. — log hop/ledge hop)
④ Over a landscaping timber (T.E. — log hop)
⑤ Up the curb into garden (T.E. — ascending rocky stairsteps)
⑥ Over the garden wall into driveway (T.E. — going off a medium drop-off)
⑦ Over the landscaping timber (T.E. — log hop)
⑧ Up the steps (T.E. — Ascending a large rockpile)
⑨ Off the porch (T.E. — going off a big ledge)
⑩ Whacked in the face by an angry spouse or spousal equivalent. (T.E.: encountering an extremely hostile landowner or intractable ranger, $T.E.^2$: having a really bad crash!

65

The Basic Moves

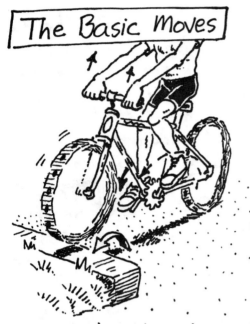

Front Wheel Hop - This is lifting the front wheel by pulling up on the bars combined with a hard pedal stroke in a low gear. The Front Wheel Hop is the foundation move for the wheelie, wheelie hop, log hop and the pivot turn. Concentrate on bringing the cranks level after the pedal stroke to avoid ground clutter and to set up for dyno-moves.

Front Wheel Hop + Rear Wheel Lift - After the front wheel is raised, bounce upward from level cranks and punch the bars forward, raising the rear wheel (at least, theo-retically). Add energy to the bounce and a bar punch, and you've got the rudimentary "Wheelie Hop".

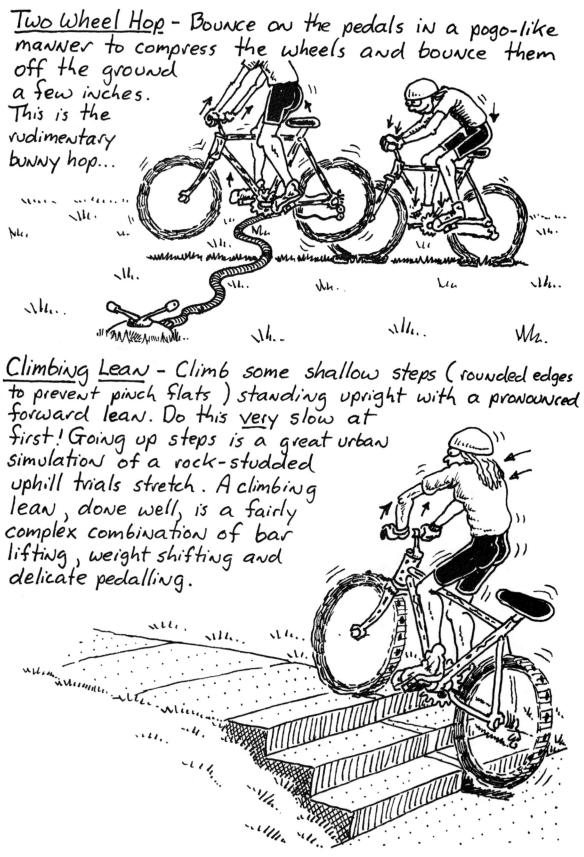

Two Wheel Hop – Bounce on the pedals in a pogo-like manner to compress the wheels and bounce them off the ground a few inches. This is the rudimentary bunny hop...

Climbing Lean – Climb some shallow steps (rounded edges to prevent pinch flats) standing upright with a pronounced forward lean. Do this <u>very</u> slow at first! Going up steps is a great urban simulation of a rock-studded uphill trials stretch. A climbing lean, done well, is a fairly complex combination of bar lifting, weight shifting and delicate pedalling.

Rear Lean Move - Go off a small drop standing, fluidly moving your torso behind the seat then back up on landing. Go very slow at first, concentrating on a smooth weight transfer. Move to higher and higher speeds and add an upward pull to the bars as you cross the lip of the drop so you land on both wheels simultaneously. For really mushy landing spots, add more bar lift so you land rear wheel first!

Whoaaaaa!

Front Wheel Aerial Lift - Find a rounded hump or small upgrade with a soft grassy runout. You can ride off this obstacle several ways at different speeds to simulate a variety of on trail dyno-moves;

1. Hit the hump standing (legs "flexed") and lift the bars at the crest. You should get some moderate air time and land with both wheels hitting the ground simultaneously. Be sure to get in the habit of absorbing landing shock in the legs, not the arms. This applies particularly when you're landing on loose or mushy ground... the front wheel must be held firmly to keep it from turning sideways on landing.

68

2. Hit the hump standing, at moderate speed, and dyno-relax your arms and legs on contact. You should not get air and your head should remain level. This is "passive bump swallowing." The upward motion of the bike on contact with the hump bounces the bike over the obstacle...

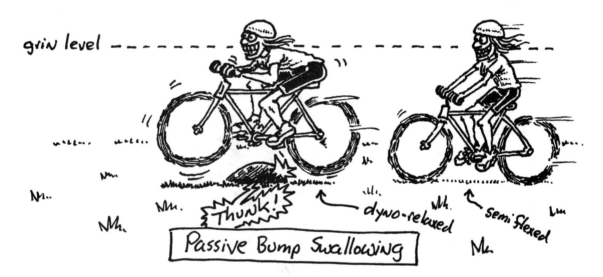

grin level

Thunk!

dyno-relaxed   semi-flexed

Passive Bump Swallowing

2. (contd.) Now approach the hump again at moderate speed. Let the hump compress the tires, setting up a bunny hop. Instead of relaxing to absorb shock, you are maximizing the shock and following thru with an upward lunge at "deadpoint" to raise the bike higher.

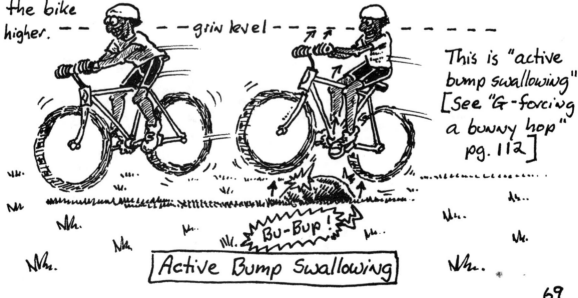

grin level

This is "active bump swallowing" [See "G-forcing a bunny hop" pg. 112]

Bu-Bup!

Active Bump Swallowing

③ Now for some massive air time... hit the hump "flexed" in a pre-hop coil. As the front wheel hits the top of the hump, uncoil your body and jerk the bars upward. You can skip the pre-hop bounce because being "flexed" (no shock absorbed by legs & arms) causes "dyno-compression" of both wheels and, combined with the bar jerk, yields tons of up-energy for serious flight time. The harder and faster you hit the hump, the higher and farther you fly [See: "G-Forcing a Bunny Hop" pg. 112] Once you've honed this move sequence, consider adding an inflight bar lift (done by merely rolling back with the wrists) so's you don't land front wheel first and get splattered!

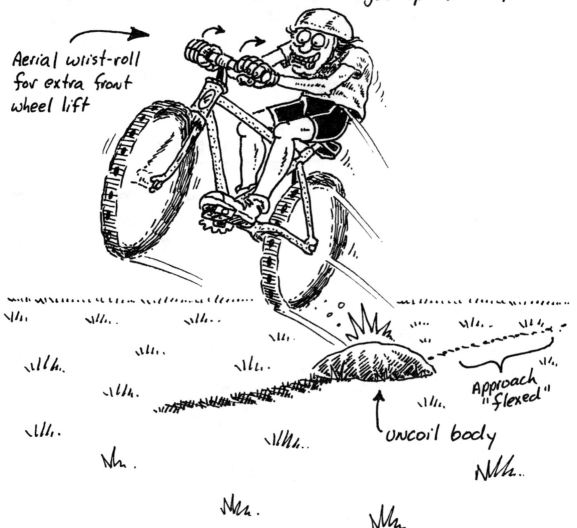

Aerial wrist-roll for extra front wheel lift

Approach "flexed"

uncoil body

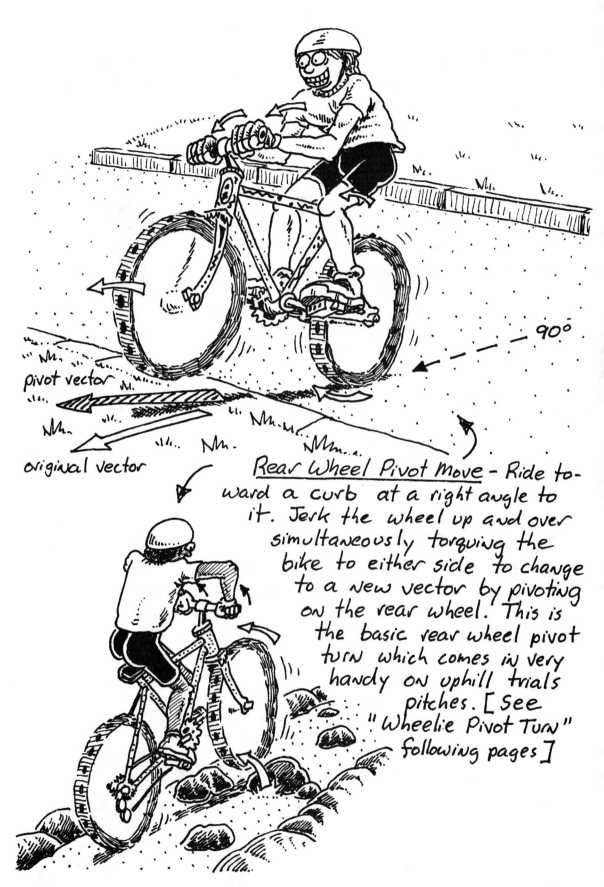

90°

pivot vector

original vector

Rear Wheel Pivot Move - Ride toward a curb at a right angle to it. Jerk the wheel up and over simultaneously torquing the bike to either side to change to a new vector by pivoting on the rear wheel. This is the basic rear wheel pivot turn which comes in very handy on uphill trials pitches. [See "Wheelie Pivot Turn" following pages]

Skid Moves

Skid Moves – Find some soft ground and ride across it at **moderate speed**. Lock the rear wheel and lean in the direction you wish to turn. You should slide 90° around the front wheel pivot point ending perpendicular to your original direction. Add control by using some front brake "let-offs" and a harder lean.

All skid moves can have a negative impact on the trail environment so be aware when using them! You can minimize skid move impact by keeping your speed down whenever you do one.

Braked Descending

Braked Descending   Ideally a series of skid moves without the "skid." Great for going down way-gnarly twisting staircase pitches. You want to start ultra-slow and slowly bounce your way down. Keep your rear wheel semi-locked and maintain control by selectively adding and letting-off pressure on the front brake pads. Lock the front wheel and you'll do an ultra-nasty head dab! Needless to say, start with very easy down-pitches until you master the complex interplay of rear leaning, selective front braking and body torquing.

Rear Brake: 3 or 4 fingers →

Front Brake: two or thwee fingers

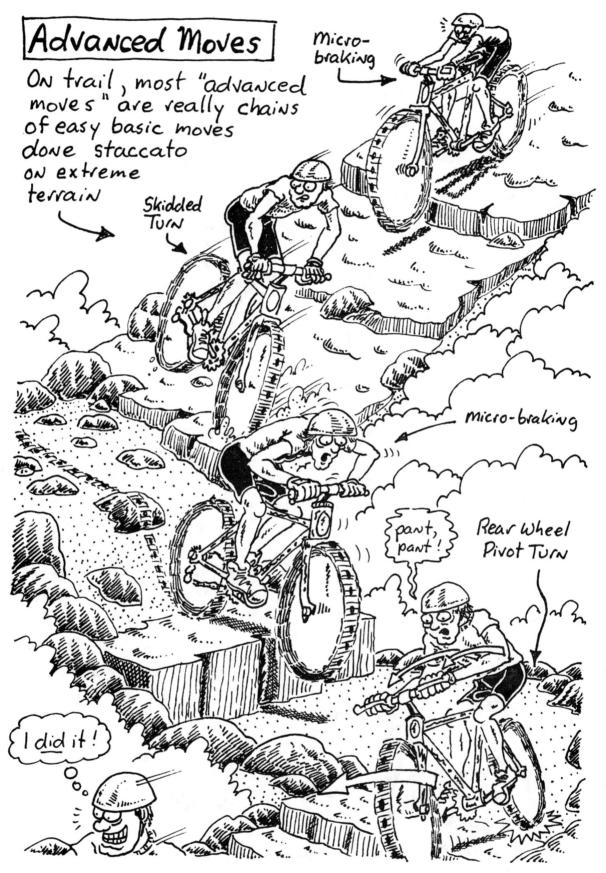

73

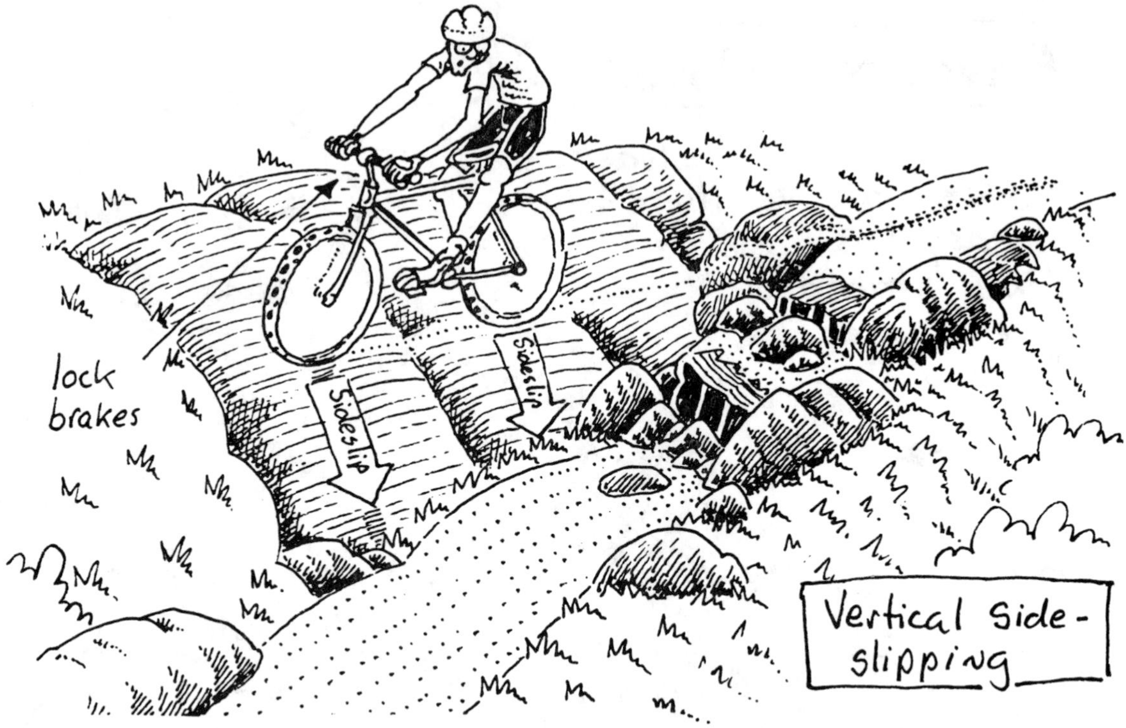

lock
brakes

Sideslip

Sideslip

Vertical Side-
slipping

<u>Vertical Side-slipping</u> - a controlled sideways skidding descent. Above, the rider continues level to bypass an obstacle with serious face-plant potential onto the highside of the trail. Locking both wheels, he slides back onto the trail, letting off on either brake lever to maintain momentum and control. Eco-hazard, use on rock only (except in dire emergencies)!

<u>Wheelie Pivot Turn</u> - This move allows a rider to make up to a 90° turn in half the length of the bike. Usually done in a semi-seated stance, a wheelie pivot turn works best on an upgrade.

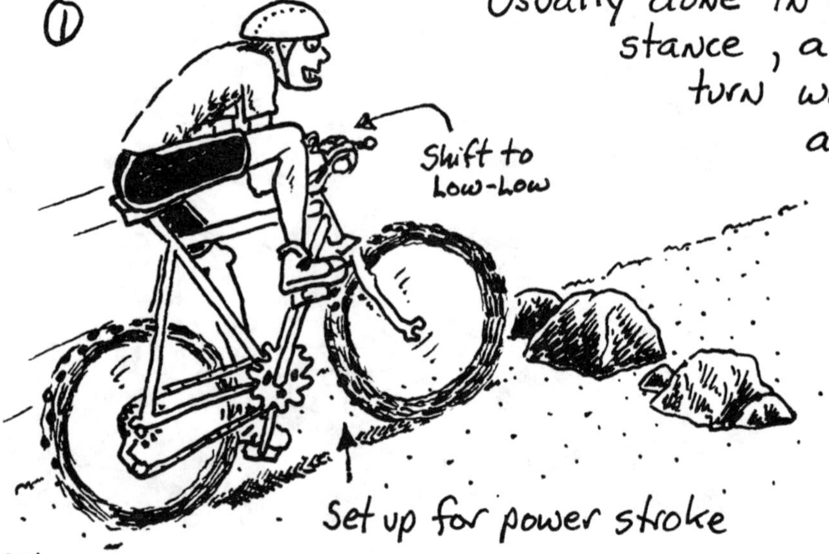

①

Shift to
Low-Low

Set up for power stroke

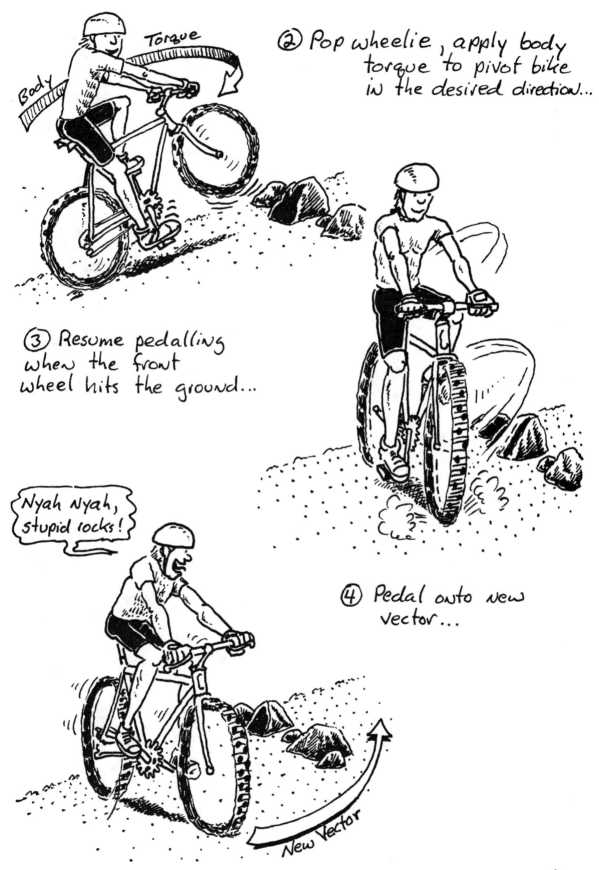

② Pop wheelie, apply body torque to pivot bike in the desired direction...

③ Resume pedalling when the front wheel hits the ground...

Nyah Nyah, stupid rocks!

④ Pedal onto new vector...

Front Wheel Skidded Turn - This is a tricky move used to cross the fall line in control while descending. Perfect for decreasing radius turns and super-tight switchbacks where an inside lean is contraindicated. One of the ultimate tests of braking and leaning techniques, here the rider endeavors to lock the front wheel on a steep downgrade and swing the rear wheel 90° around it, all without going over the bars (bottom rt.)!

Front Wheel Skidded Turn

Fall Line

This is a behind-the-seat move done on the edge of control so use caution attempting it. Obviously, like all skidded moves, it's an eco-hazard so use it accordingly.

Aiiieee!

Botched Front Wheel Skidded Turn

76

① Slow bike, get behind seat...

② Quickly lock rear wheel & rotate front wheel across the fall line and lock front brake. Release rear brake and pivot around front wheel.

Fall Line

(whew!)

Fall Line

Woosh!

front wheel almost perpendicular to frame

Using A Front Wheel Skid On trail

③ Release both brakes after pivot.

Micro-Braking -
This is a specialized & subtle braking technique usually done during slow trialsesque descending.

clickity clickity click

Both brakes are applied alternately and together for brief instants of time to do skid turns, negotiate drops or set up dyno-moves. "Let Offs" (quick brake lever releases) give you the equivalent of micro-bursts of power to do wheel hops or roll over protruding rocks/roots without having to rotate the cranks in ground cluttered conditions. A front brake let off going onto a bump will compress the tire to set you up for a hop or pivot turn without your having to jerk the bars to lift the front wheel. Like most complex riding techniques, micro-braking takes lots of practice on-trail to master.

77

Advanced Log Hopping : There are three good methods for hopping fallen logs; I."Frontpointing" (the easiest), II. Slow Wheelie Hop (next easiest), and III. the Fast Wheelie Hop (most difficult).

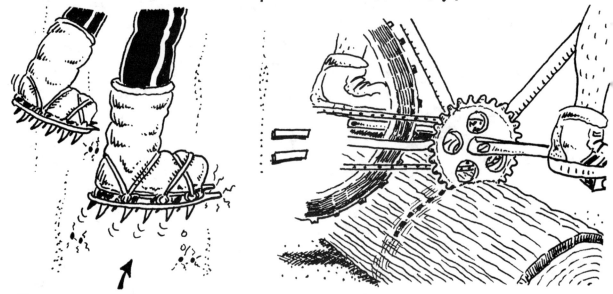

I. Frontpointing involves popping a wheelie, hitting the log and using the large chainring as a third wheel to roll over the log. This is a slo-mo move and the author suggests removing your seat while learning it...

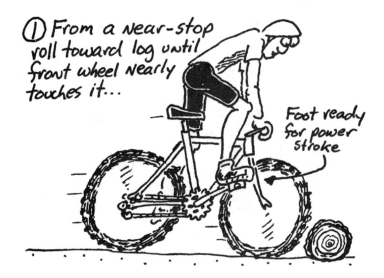

① From a near-stop roll toward log until front wheel nearly touches it...

Foot ready for power stroke

② Execute a front wheelie and roll forward on rear wheel until chainring hits log...

Be ready for hard frame shock when chain ring meets log!

Watch out for seat!

③ Stick chainring into log. If you're going too fast and/or if you've forgotten to lower the seat you will now be in great pain...

Thunk!

④ Continue pedalling and rock frame over top of log. ⟶

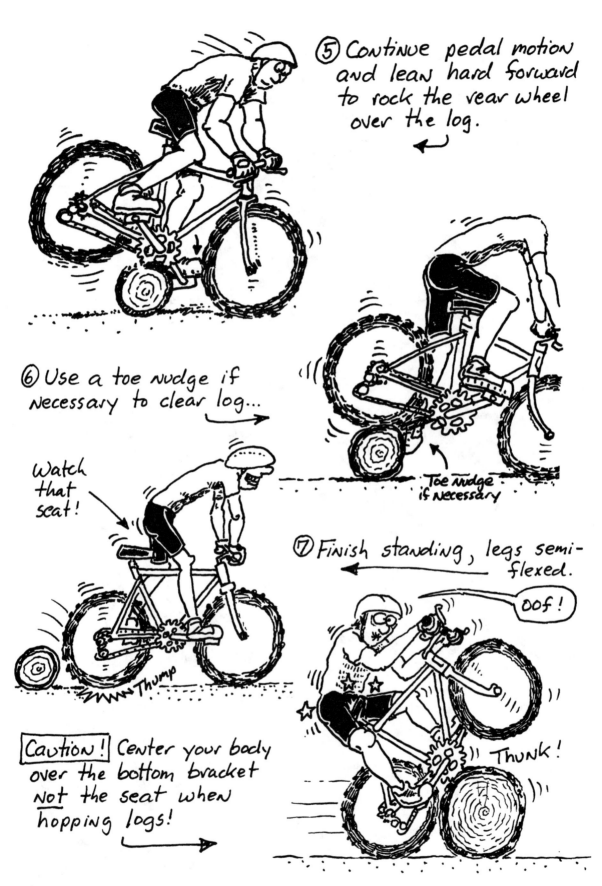

⑤ Continue pedal motion and lean hard forward to rock the rear wheel over the log.

⑥ Use a toe nudge if necessary to clear log...

Toe nudge if necessary

Watch that seat!

Thump

⑦ Finish standing, legs semi-flexed.

Oof!

Thunk!

Caution! Center your body over the bottom bracket NOT the seat when hopping logs!

II. Slow Wheelie Hop... Similar to the frontpointing method except you try not to contact the log with the chainwheel, rotating around the front wheel hub instead. The Slow Wheelie Hop requires a minor dyno-move in steps ② and ③.

① Pop wheelie...

② Level your cranks, lean forward and bunny hop...

pre-hop compression

③ As you come up into deadpoint (weight off bike) shove hard forward on the bars to bring the rear wheel up and over the log...

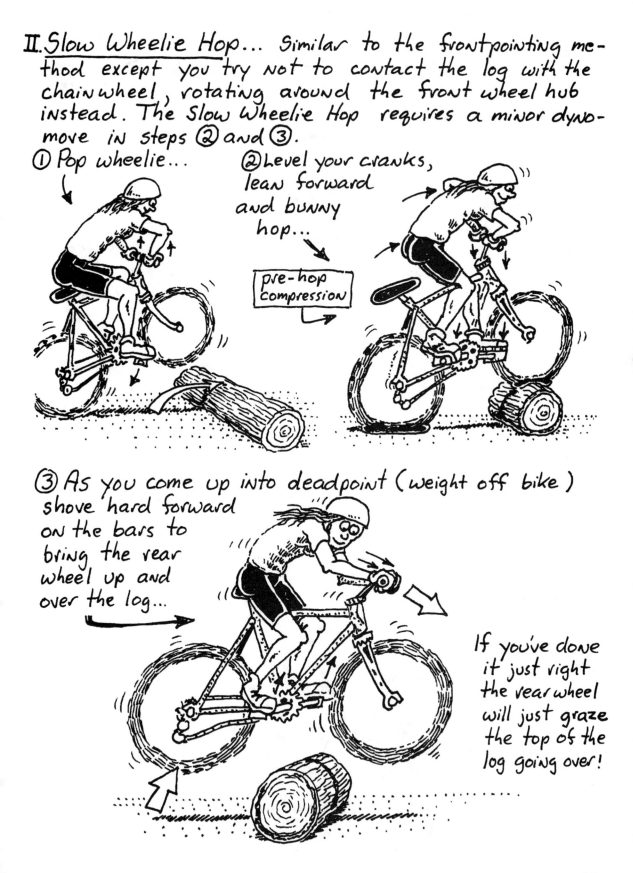

If you've done it just right the rear wheel will just graze the top of the log going over!

III. Fast Wheelie Hop – Just like the slow method only you leave out contacting the log with the front wheel, rotating in the air instead. This is an expert-level dynomove requiring serious commitment as the log is approached relatively fast... if you screw up, you're gonna get hammered!

① Approach log at moderate to high speed & execute a wheelie...

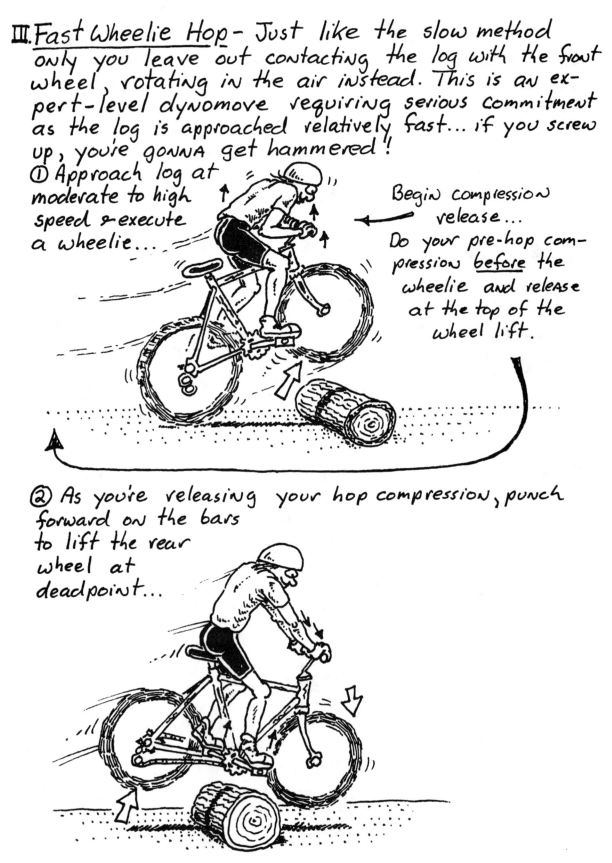

Begin compression release...

Do your pre-hop compression **before** the wheelie and release at the top of the wheel lift.

② As you're releasing your hop compression, punch forward on the bars to lift the rear wheel at deadpoint...

③ Land on front wheel using your arms to absorb shock so's you don't do a face-plant (see below).

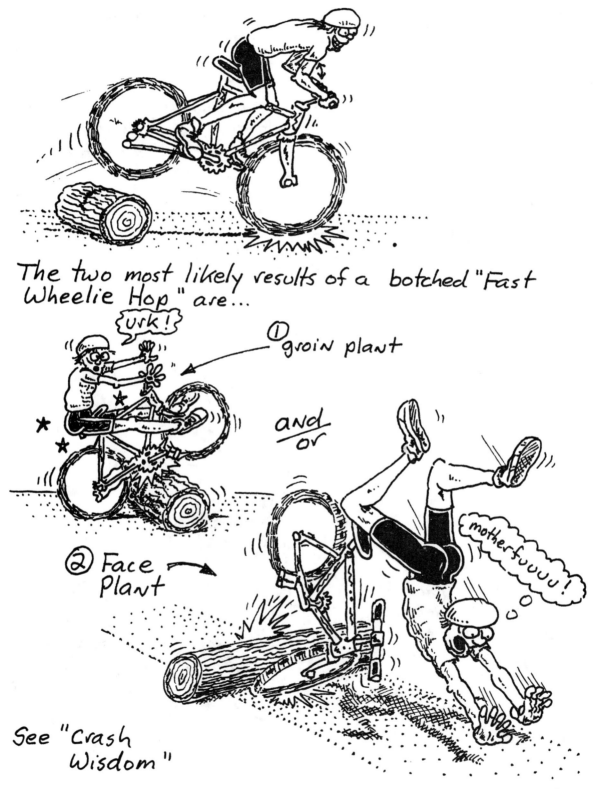

The two most likely results of a botched "Fast Wheelie Hop" are...

urk!

① groin plant

and
or

② Face Plant →

motherfuuuu!

See "Crash Wisdom"

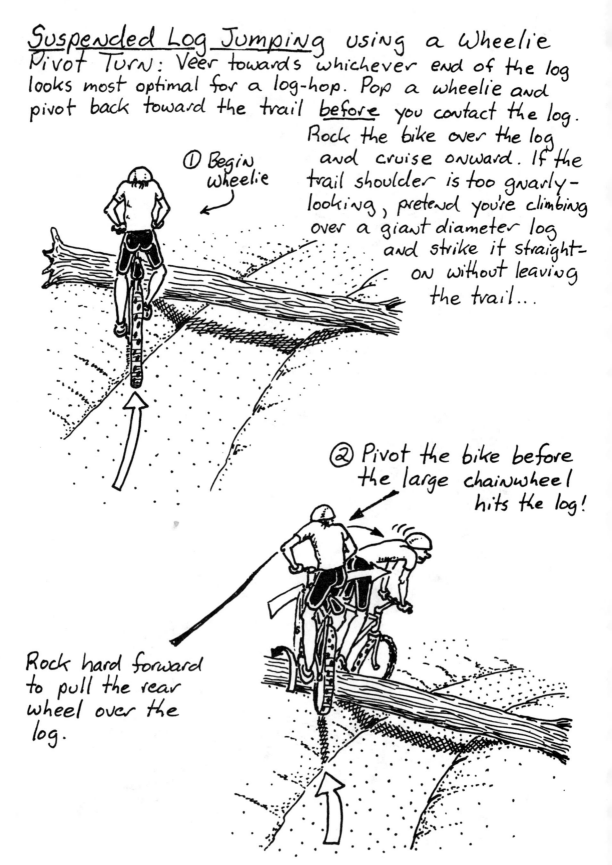

Suspended Log Jumping using a Wheelie

Pivot Turn: Veer towards whichever end of the log looks most optimal for a log-hop. Pop a wheelie and pivot back toward the trail <u>before</u> you contact the log. Rock the bike over the log and cruise onward. If the trail shoulder is too gnarly-looking, pretend you're climbing over a giant diameter log and strike it straight-on without leaving the trail...

① Begin wheelie

② Pivot the bike before the large chainwheel hits the log!

Rock hard forward to pull the rear wheel over the log.

Diagonal Log Jumping

① Crossing a diagonal log straight on will typically hang the rear wheel & the bike will slide across the face of the log...

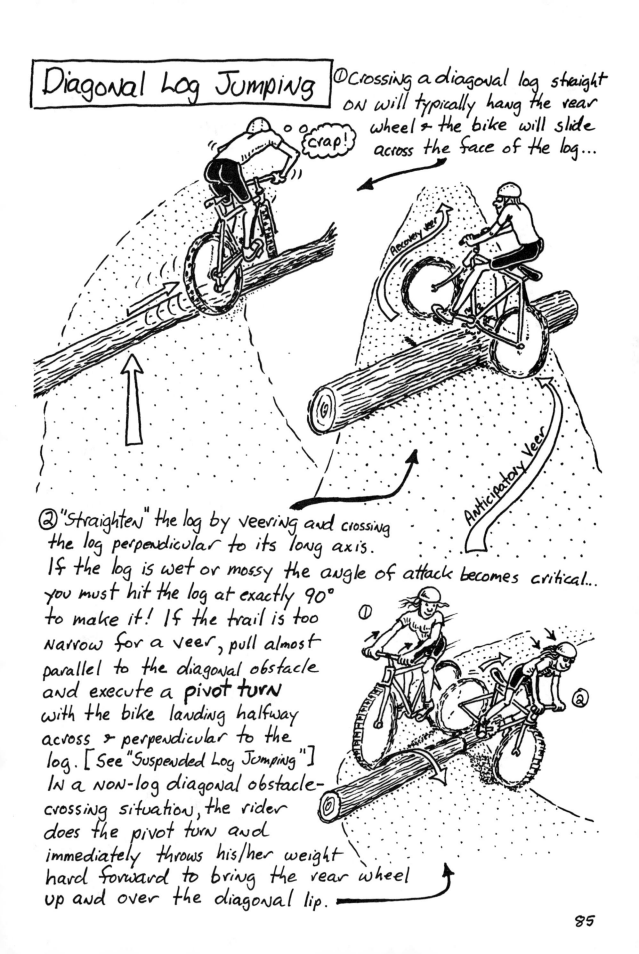

crap!

Recovery veer

Anticipatory Veer

② "Straighten" the log by veering and crossing the log perpendicular to its long axis. If the log is wet or mossy the angle of attack becomes critical... you must hit the log at exactly 90° to make it! If the trail is too narrow for a veer, pull almost parallel to the diagonal obstacle and execute a **pivot turn** with the bike landing halfway across & perpendicular to the log. [See "Suspended Log Jumping"] In a NON-log diagonal obstacle-crossing situation, the rider does the pivot turn and immediately throws his/her weight hard forward to bring the rear wheel up and over the diagonal lip.

① ②

Advanced Bunny Hop...

While the bunny hop could be called a "basic move," it requires advanced skills to do properly. It is the foundation that most on-trail dyno-moves are built upon. The bunny hop consists of two basic motion components: ① dynamically coiling the body while simultaneously compressing both wheels (fig.1) and ② Unloading (releasing) the compressed tires and springing upward to deadpoint (fig.2).

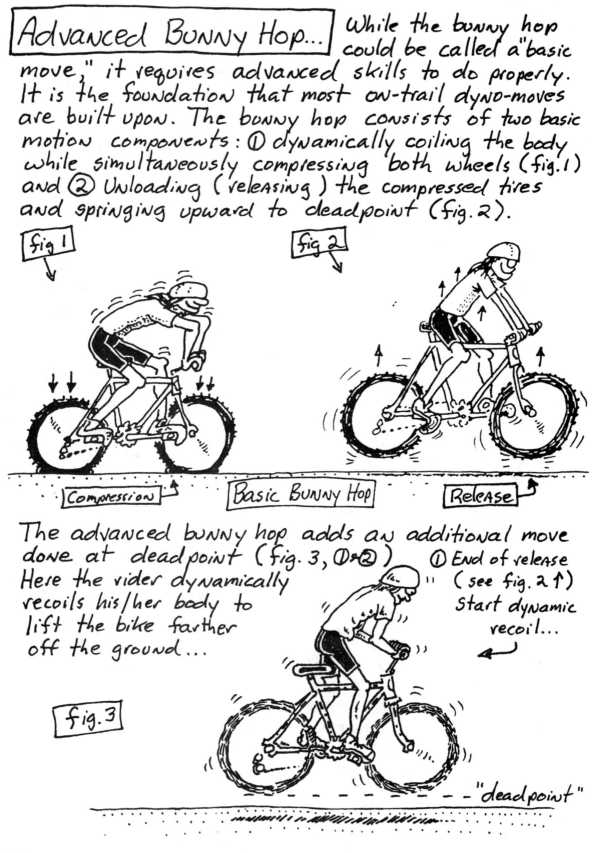

fig 1

fig 2

Compression   Basic Bunny Hop   Release

The advanced bunny hop adds an additional move done at deadpoint (fig. 3, ①&②) Here the rider dynamically recoils his/her body to lift the bike farther off the ground...

① End of release (see fig. 2 ↑) Start dynamic recoil...

fig. 3

"deadpoint"

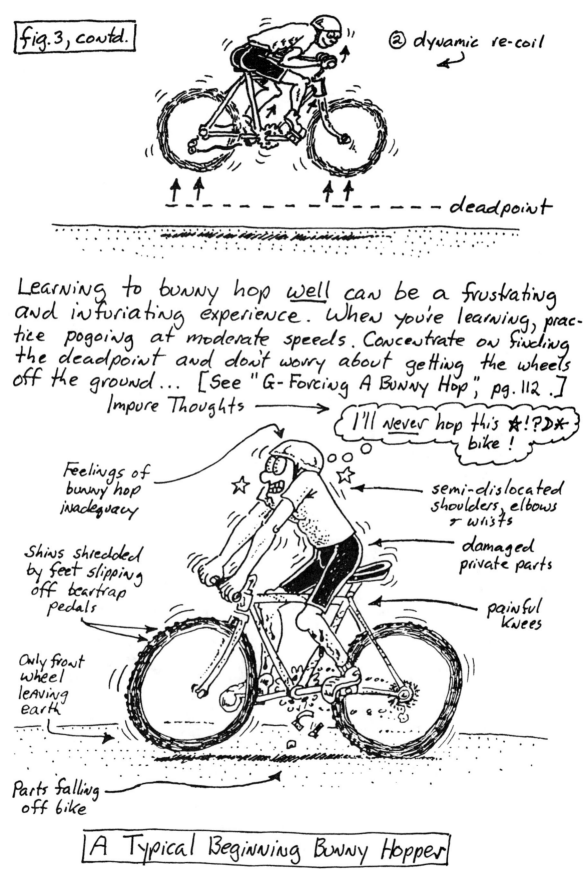

② dynamic re-coil

deadpoint

Learning to bunny hop <u>well</u> can be a frustrating and infuriating experience. When you're learning, practice pogoing at moderate speeds. Concentrate on finding the deadpoint and don't worry about getting the wheels off the ground... [See "G-Forcing A Bunny Hop", pg. 112.]

Impure Thoughts →

I'll <u>never</u> hop this *!?D* bike!

Feelings of bunny hop inadequacy

semi-dislocated shoulders, elbows & wrists

damaged private parts

Shins shredded by feet slipping off beartrap pedals

painful knees

Only front wheel leaving earth

Parts falling off bike

A Typical Beginning Bunny Hopper

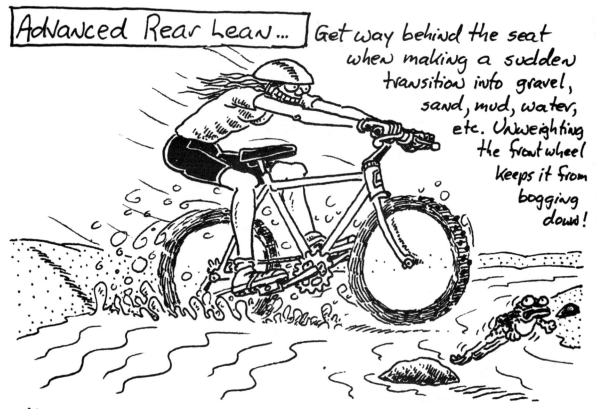

Advanced Rear Lean... Get way behind the seat when making a sudden transition into gravel, sand, mud, water, etc. Unweighting the front wheel keeps it from bogging down!

Also move behind the seat on precipitous down-grades and don't forget to move forward when you bottom-out and start uphill!

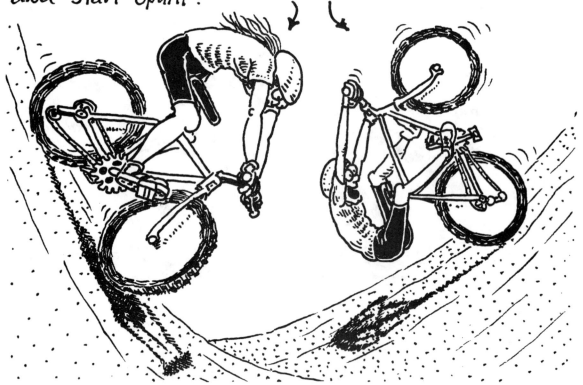

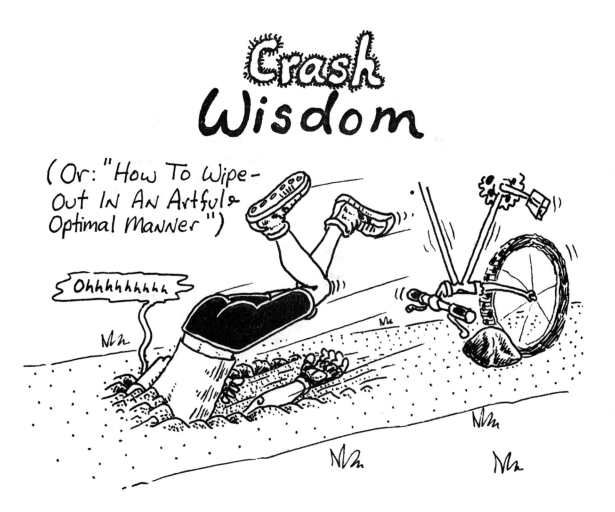

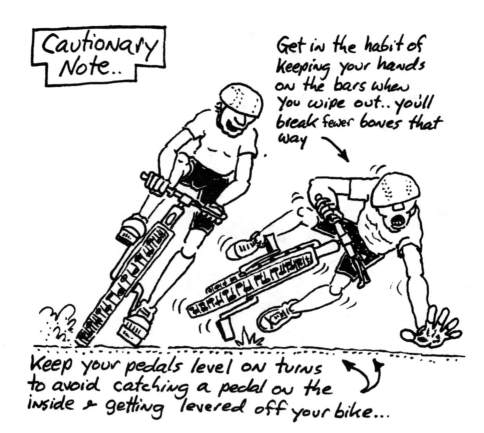

Cautionary Note..

Get in the habit of keeping your hands on the bars when you wipe out.. you'll break fewer bones that way

Keep your pedals level on turns to avoid catching a pedal on the inside & getting levered off your bike...

Learning To Fall...

One of the first things you'll notice about beginning mtn. biking is, if you ride in a normal self-challenging manner, you will be taking a _lot_ of falls initially.

If you want to survive the novice level with a minimum of injuries, it's best to acknowledge falldom & learn to fall artfully, ie: in a non-injurious & graceful manner. As your riding competance increases, falls will become relatively infrequent although my experience has shown that what advanced level falls lack in frequency is made up in sheer bone-crunching, swatted-by-the-entire-planet energy. The better you ride, the faster you go, the harder you fall. Learning good fall technique at the beginning will benefit you throughout your mtn. biking career!

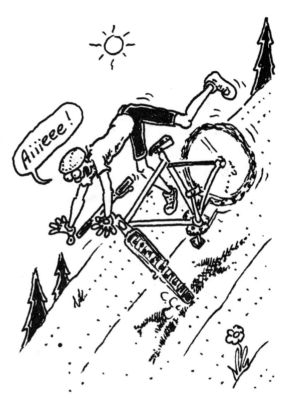

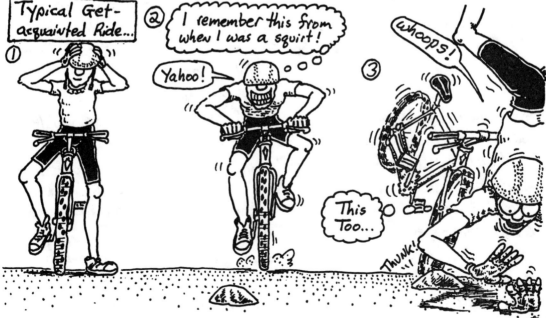

Typical Get-acquainted Ride...
①
② "I remember this from when I was a squirt!" "Yahoo!"
③ "Whoops!" "This Too..." THUNK!

Aiiieee!

The best way to prevent mtn. bike-related injuries is to leave the bike chained-up in the carport and watch golf on TV. Riding like a twit (conservatively) will also cut down on accidents (fig. 1) but where's the fun in that !?

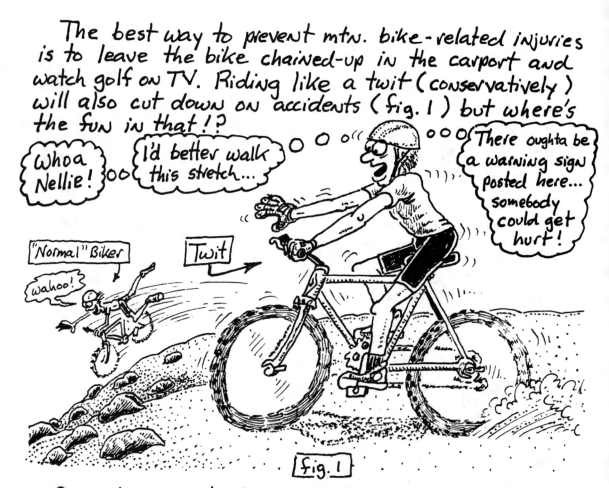

Whoa Nellie!

I'd better walk this stretch...

There oughta be a warning sign posted here... somebody could get hurt!

"Normal" Biker

wahoo!

Twit

fig. 1

Since the object of mtn. biking is to have way too much fun without paying too dearly for it, most of us ride like maniacs at the very edge of control (where politically correct). Thus, wipe-outs are relatively normal. How the rider reacts in a crash situation will pretty much determine the seriousness of a given crash.

Think of mtn. biking as a martial art of the defensive variety like Judo. One of the first things you learn in Judo is how to hit the mat hard and quickly recover without getting hurt. Sneak into a gym with a wrestling mat and learn how to fall. Concentrate on the "running front flip" which simulates the dreaded (and common) over-the-bars body slam, the most potentially injurious mtn. bike accident-type (fig. 2). In a low-speed trials-type over-the-bars front flip you may elect to let go of the bars and do a rolling vault off well-flexed arms

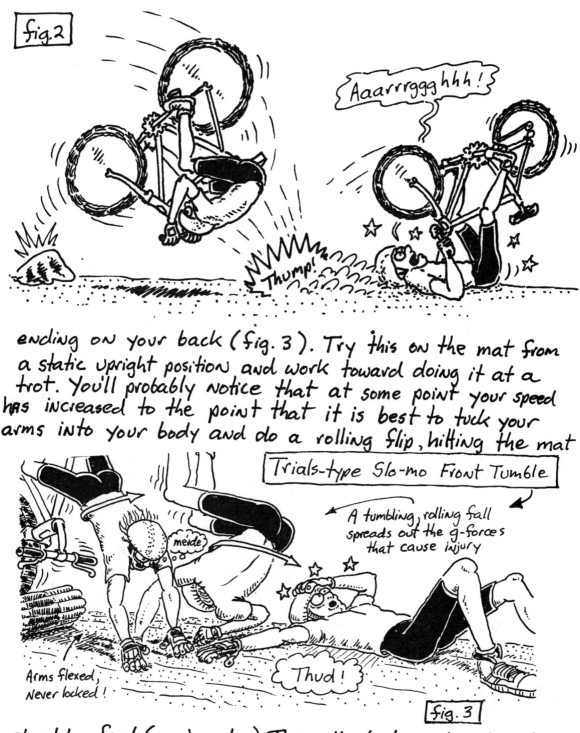

fig.2

Aaarrrgggghhh!

Thump!

ending on your back (fig. 3). Try this on the mat from a static upright position and work toward doing it at a trot. You'll probably notice that at some point your speed has increased to the point that it is best to tuck your arms into your body and do a rolling flip, hitting the mat

Trials-type Slo-mo Front Tumble

A tumbling, rolling fall spreads out the g-forces that cause injury

merde

Arms flexed, Never locked!

Thud!

fig. 3

shoulder first (no hands). This illustrates why it is best to keep your hands on the bars in a moderate to high speed crash: if you don't you'll probably break both arms then land on your head (fig 6)! Practice running, front-flipping and rolling without using your arms, on a mat (fig. 4). You will know you've got it down when Ⓐ it doesn't hurt much anymore, and ⑥ you're ending upright in a low crouch. This is what you want to happen when you go over the bars

fig. 4

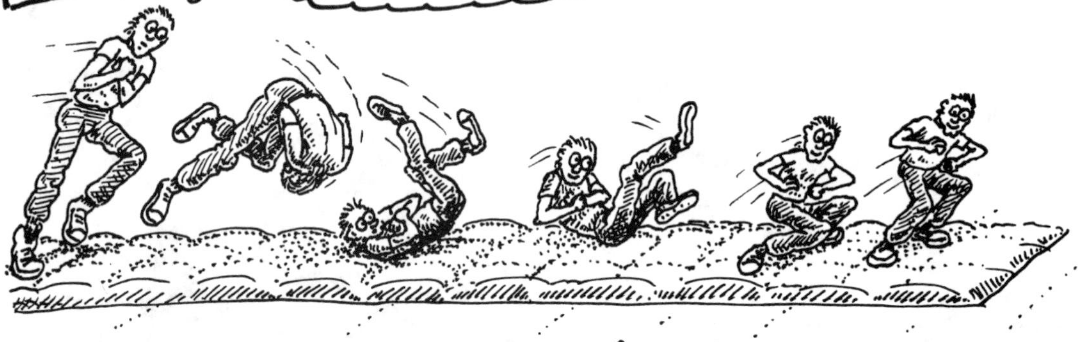

This is In-sane!

at moderate to high speeds (fig. 5). When you go over the bars at high speed you **will do a front flip!** The trick is developing the discipline to tuck your head, bend your back, hang onto the bars and roll with it (see figs. 5 & 6). If you don't you will get hurt, perhaps seriously!

fig. 5

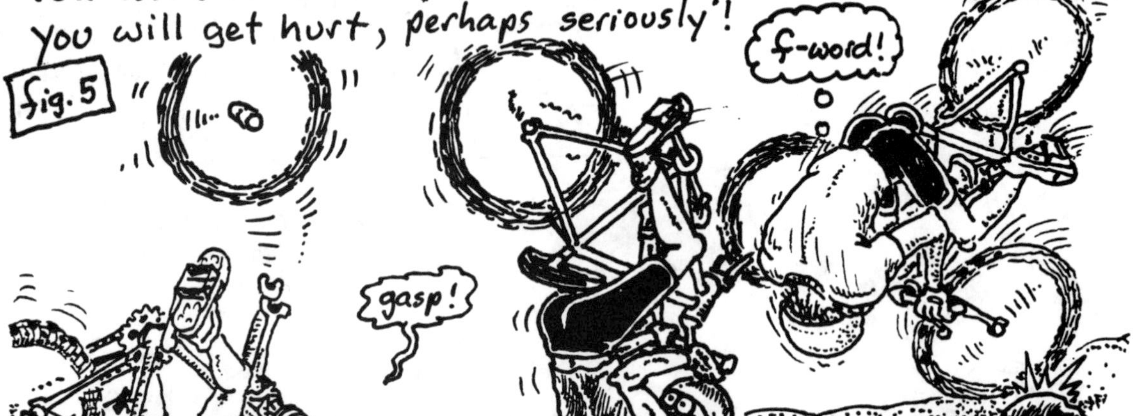

f-word!

gasp!

Oof!

fig. 6 What happens if you try to catch a high-speed fall with your arms....

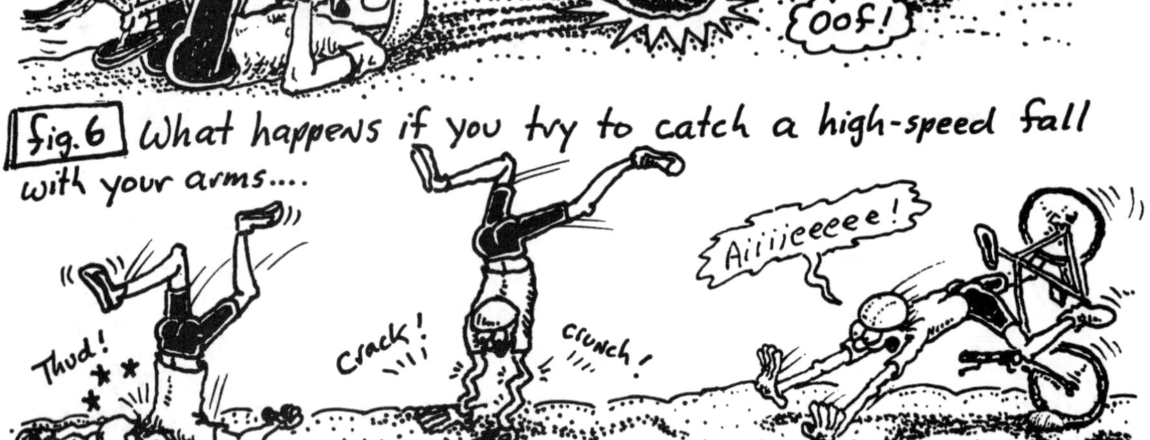

Thud! * *

Crack!

Crunch!

Aiiiieeeee!

Another excellent reason to hang onto your bike in any fall is a loose bike's proclivity to become a very gnarly projectile during a wipe-out!

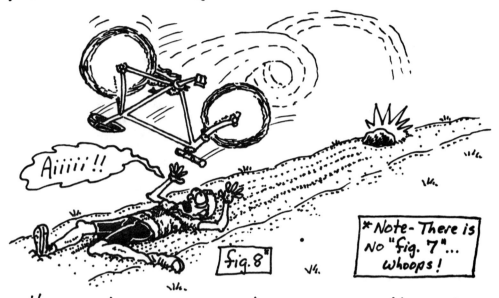

Aiiiii!!

fig.8*

*Note - There is NO "fig. 7"... whoops!

The other most common crash scenario is the sideways fall. At _very_ low speeds it is probably safe to attempt to check the fall with a foot or, as a last resort, an arm. At medium to high speeds it is best to remain attached to the bike, relax and roll onto the ground. This is sort of a modified "Parachute Landing Fall" with the bike & rider hitting the ground sequentially, spreading out the shock. An ideal ground-contact sequence would be ① foot and pedal, ② calf→thigh→handlebar ③ hip→forearm→arm→shoulder. The bike itself absorbs much of the impact in the pedal/crank and the end of the handlebar. Staying connected to the bike and relaxing are the keys to a painless sideways fall at speed!

You should practice this technique on soft turf to train

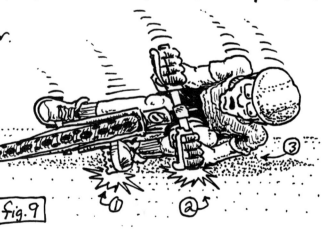

fig. 9

out the understandable tendency to check the fall with your arms.
Repeat till you're rolling onto the ground smoothly with your arms and feet remaining firmly attached to the bike.

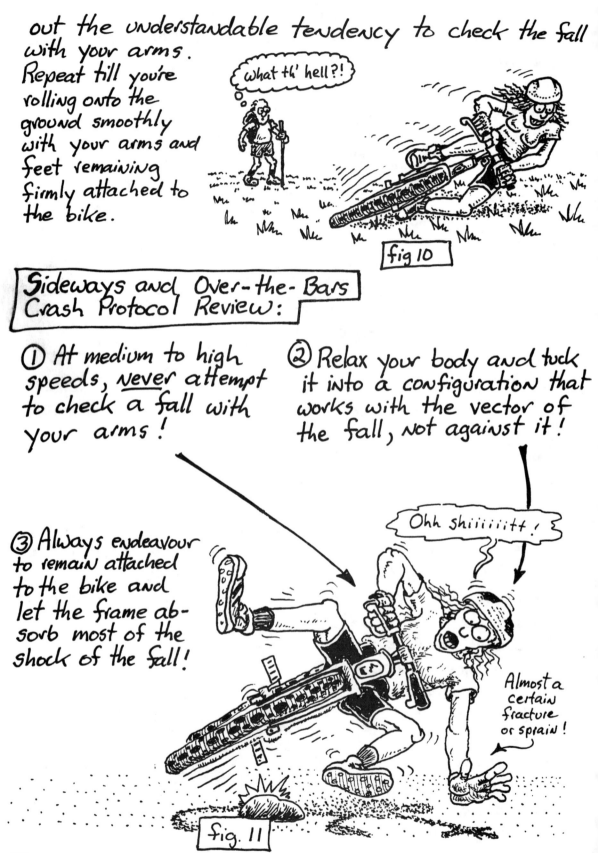

what th' hell?!

fig 10

Sideways and Over-the-Bars Crash Protocol Review:

① At medium to high speeds, <u>never</u> attempt to check a fall with your arms!

② Relax your body and tuck it into a configuration that works with the vector of the fall, not against it!

③ Always endeavour to remain attached to the bike and let the frame absorb most of the shock of the fall!

Ohh shiiiiiitt !

Almost a certain fracture or sprain!

fig. 11

A backward fall (fig.12) can be checked with the feet at any speed up to 20 mph! As the bike goes vertical, hang onto the bars, slide out of the toe clips, and basically run behind the bike which is now up on one wheel (fig.13).

This is a basic "Dynamic Dismount" (following pages). Most "dynamic dismounts" are fairly safe and can be attempted anytime <u>except</u> when the direction of the fall endangers the head, neck, or spine !!

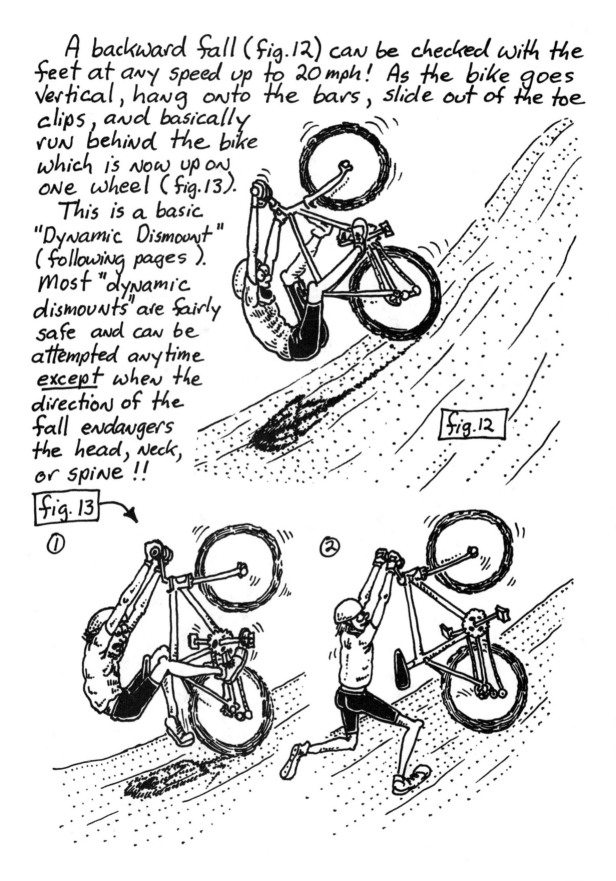

fig.12

fig.13

① ②

Dynamic Dismounts..

One great way to avoid a crash is to literally bail out before it happens. It takes practice to develop the timing so you initiate the bail-out move early enough in the developing crash. A too-late bail-out move can actually amplify crash forces!

Front Dismount

(a.k.a. "Bar Hopping") A low to medium speed step-over move to theoretically avoid a face plant. Done wrong, a bar hop almost guarantees a spectacular face plant!

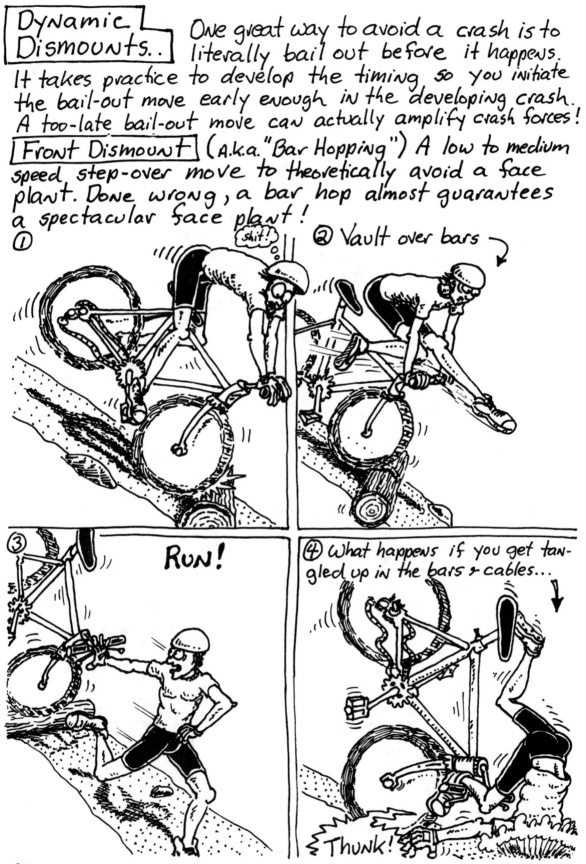

① shit!

② Vault over bars

③ RUN!

④ What happens if you get tangled up in the bars & cables... Thunk!

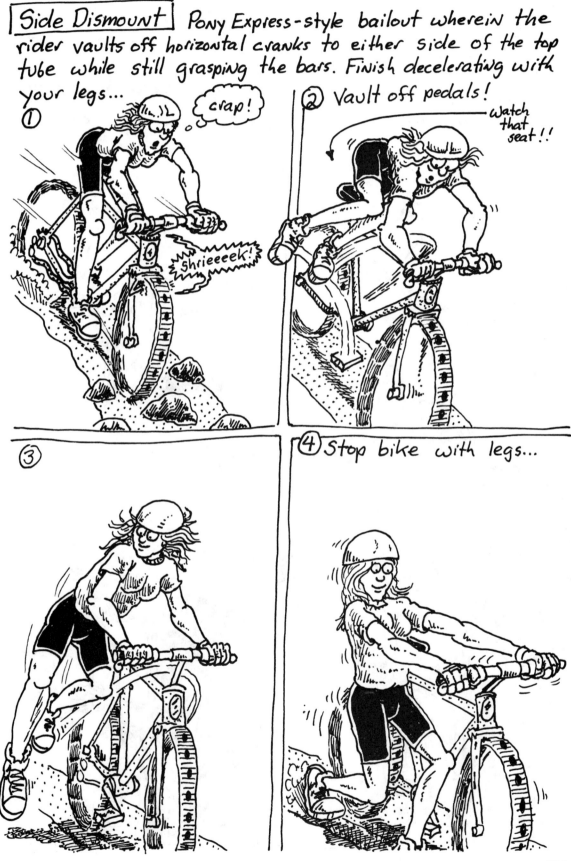

101

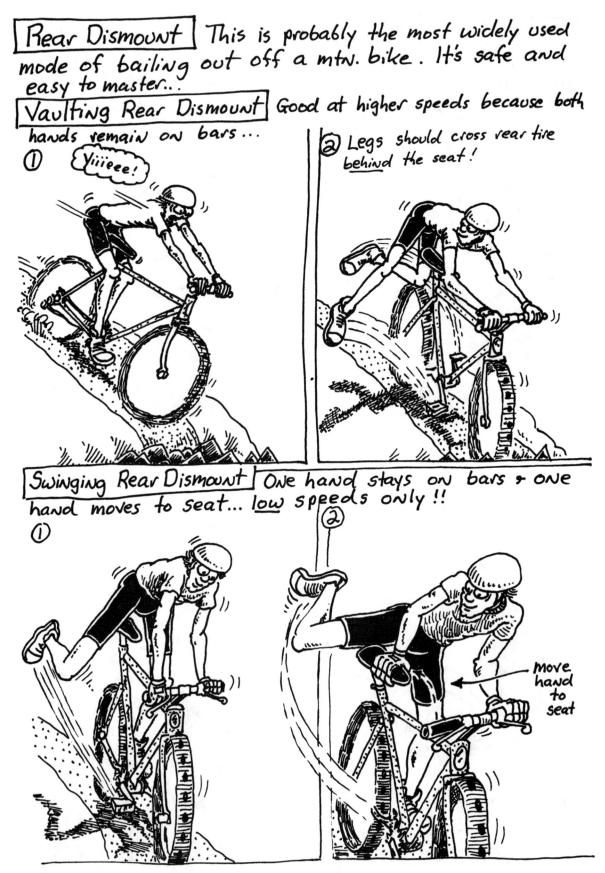

Rear Dismount This is probably the most widely used mode of bailing out off a mtn. bike. It's safe and easy to master...

Vaulting Rear Dismount Good at higher speeds because both hands remain on bars...

① *Yiiieee!*

② Legs should cross rear tire *behind* the seat!

Swinging Rear Dismount One hand stays on bars + one hand moves to seat... *low* speeds only!!

①

②

move hand to seat

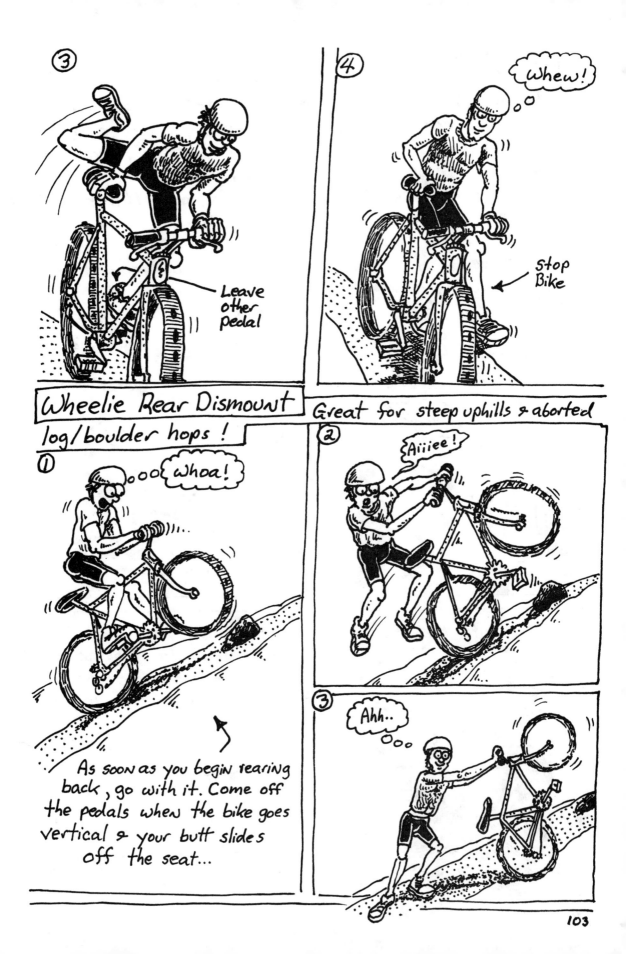

The Motorcyclist's Laydown Trick: In a truly desperate high-speed "fixing-to-crash-and-die" type situation where you know you are about to strike a pedestrian/automobile/etc. at very high speed, lock the rear brake and lay the bike down. This will quickly bleed off speed and put the bike frame between you and the obstacle. By locking the <u>rear wheel</u> you'll throw the bike into a sideways skid and avoid being launched headfirst into the obstacle. Again, stay attached to the bike & let the pedal and handlebars absorb the shock. This will also save you some skin as you skid on your side into the obstacle...

① Lock rear wheel...

ohmygod!

② Lay the bike down when sideways...

Screeeeecch!

③ Slide into the obstacle. You can use your feet to keep from going under vehicular obstacles. If it's a person or other organic obstacle at least you'll hit 'em low!

Ka-Whump!

ouchouchouchouchouchouch

fig. 10-A

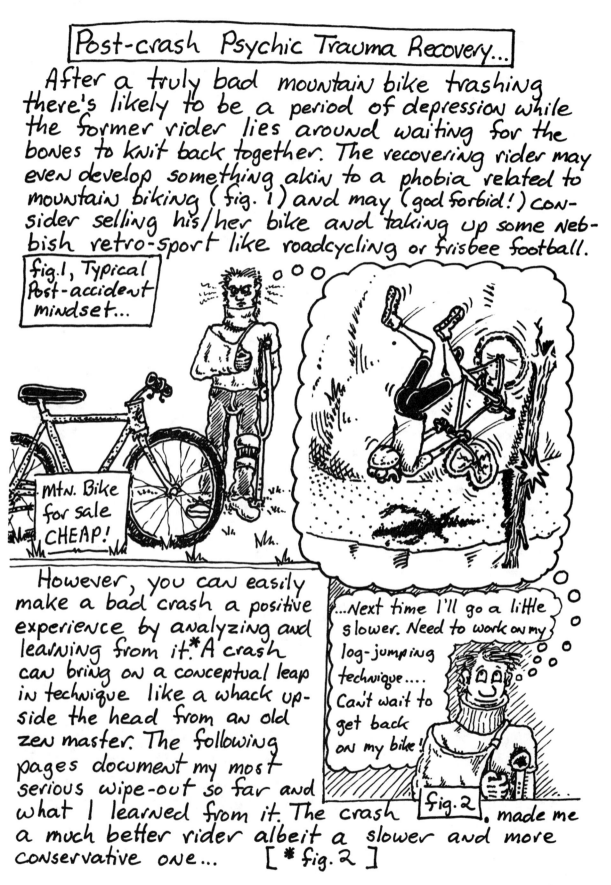

Post-crash Psychic Trauma Recovery...

After a truly bad mountain bike trashing there's likely to be a period of depression while the former rider lies around waiting for the bones to knit back together. The recovering rider may even develop something akin to a phobia related to mountain biking (fig. 1) and may (god forbid!) consider selling his/her bike and taking up some nebbish retro-sport like roadcycling or frisbee football.

fig. 1, Typical Post-accident mindset...

mtn. Bike for sale CHEAP!

However, you can easily make a bad crash a positive experience by analyzing and learning from it.* A crash can bring on a conceptual leap in technique like a whack upside the head from an old zen master. The following pages document my most serious wipe-out so far and what I learned from it. The crash made me a much better rider albeit a slower and more conservative one... [* fig. 2]

...Next time I'll go a little slower. Need to work on my log-jumping technique.... Can't wait to get back on my bike!

fig. 2

What I Learned From An Actual Crash...

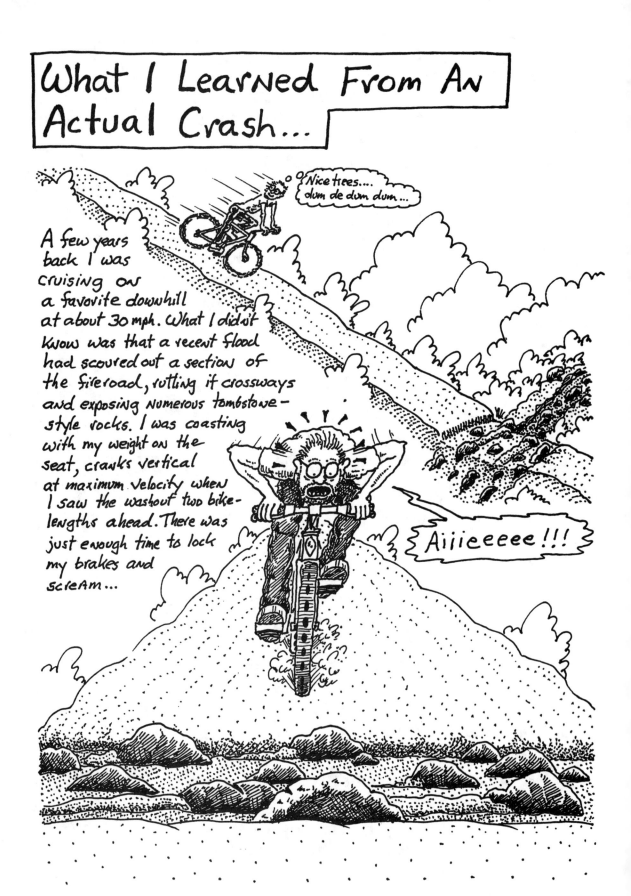

Nice trees.... dum de dum dum...

A few years back I was cruising on a favorite downhill at about 30 mph. What I didn't know was that a recent flood had scoured out a section of the fireroad, rutting it crossways and exposing numerous tombstone-style rocks. I was coasting with my weight on the seat, cranks vertical at maximum velocity when I saw the washout two bike-lengths ahead. There was just enough time to lock my brakes and scream...

Aiiieeeee!!!

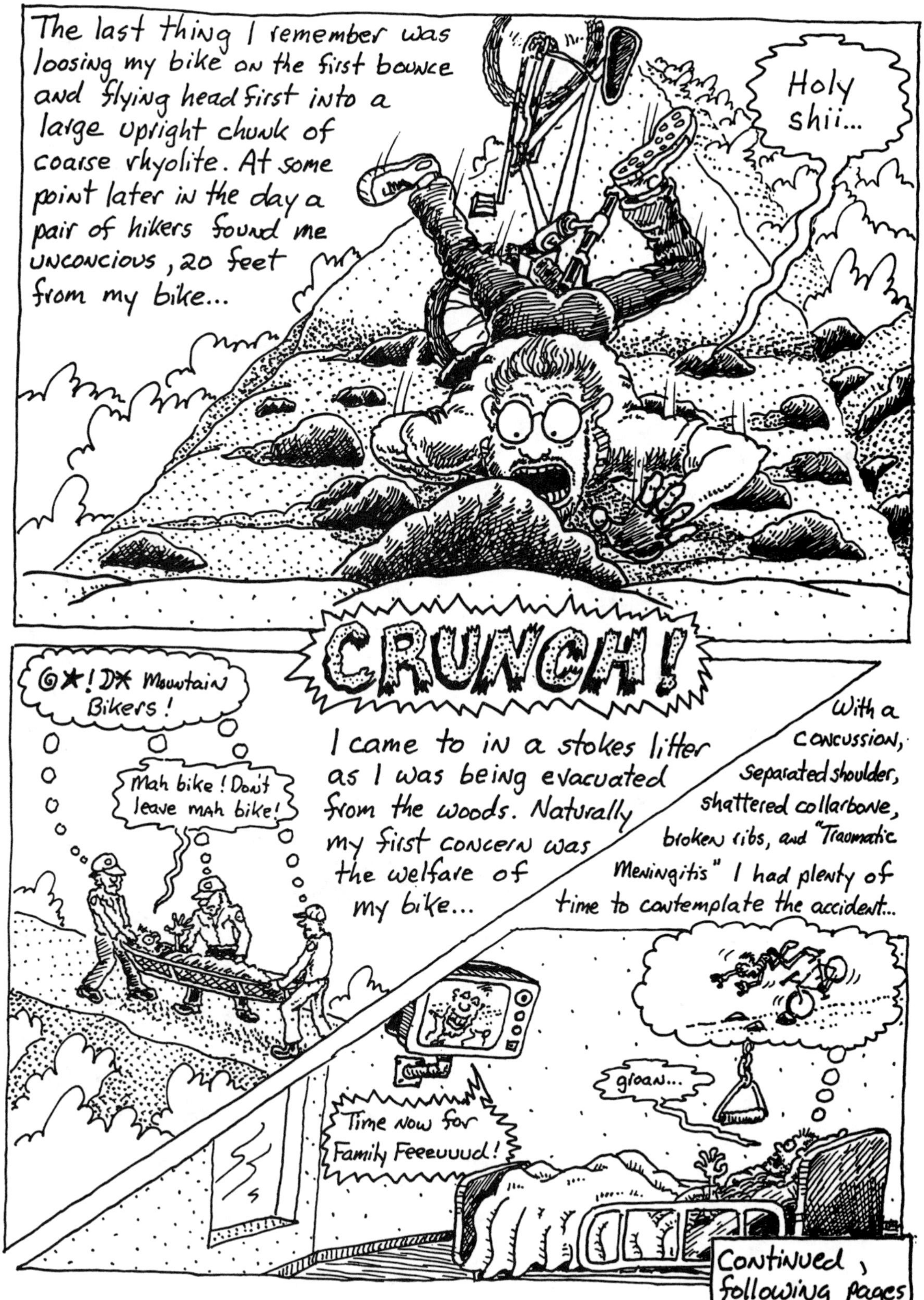

The last thing I remember was loosing my bike on the first bounce and flying head first into a large upright chunk of coarse rhyolite. At some point later in the day a pair of hikers found me unconcious, 20 feet from my bike...

Holy shii...

CRUNCH!

@*!D* Mountain Bikers!

Mah bike! Don't leave mah bike!

I came to in a stokes litter as I was being evacuated from the woods. Naturally my first concern was the welfare of my bike...

Time now for Family Feeeuuud!

gnoan...

With a concussion, separated shoulder, shattered collarbone, broken ribs, and "Traumatic Meningitis" I had plenty of time to contemplate the accident...

Continued, following pages

107

So, besides ⓐnot wearing a helmet, ⓑriding alone in a remote area, ⓒassuming trail conditions remain fixed over time, and ⓓ riding too damned fast, **WHAT** had I done technique-wise to get crashed and burned? My analysis centered on my pre-crash riding posture... I realized the way I was sitting on my bike virtually guaranteed a catastrophic rider ejection if the tires met any serious surface irregularity such as an upright rock, root, or a deep rut. I call this "ballistic posture": the rider is con- nected to the bike by gravity with no flex in his/her appendages to absorb shock.

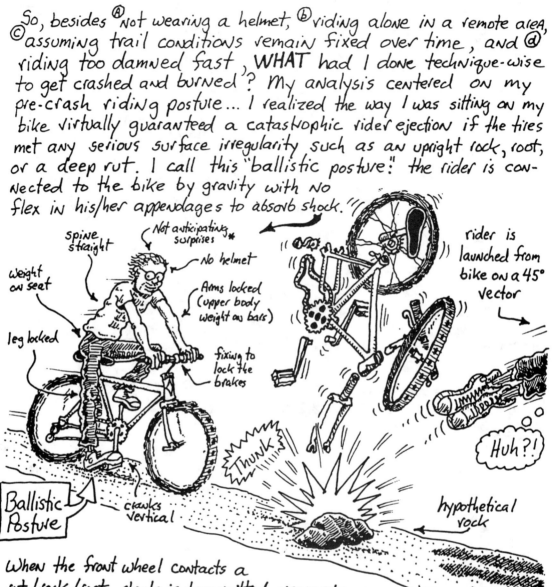

spine straight

Not anticipating surprises *

No helmet

weight on seat

Arms locked (upper body weight on bars)

leg locked

fixing to lock the brakes

rider is launched from bike on a 45° vector

Huh?!

Ballistic Posture

cranks vertical

Thunk

hypothetical rock

When the front wheel contacts a rut/rock/root, shock is transmitted upwards thru the forks and frame. If the rider's arms, spine, and legs are locked the rider has a major tendency to lose control of the bike and to be launched up and over the handlebars. Locking the brakes pre-crash only <u>adds</u> energy to the launch of the rider...

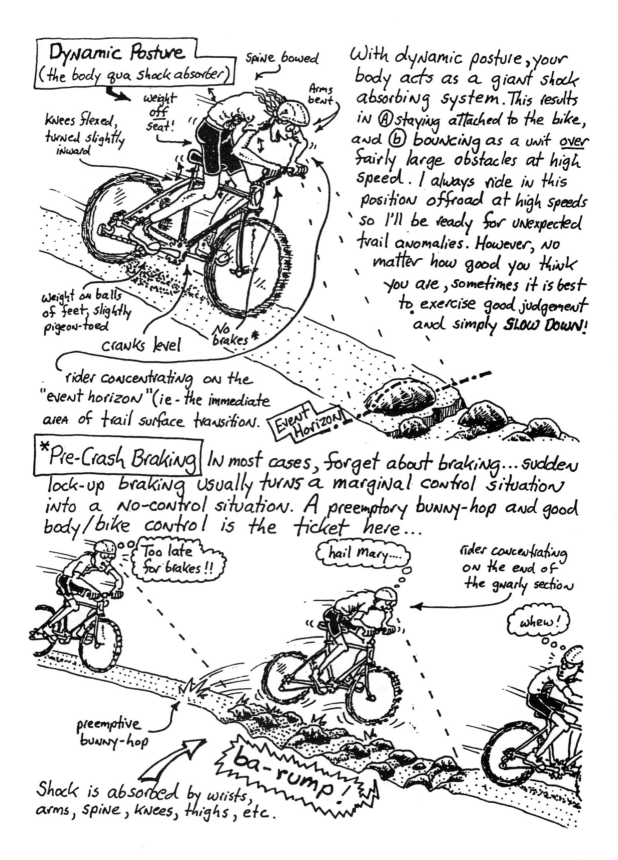

Dynamic Posture
(the body qua shock absorber)

spine bowed

Arms bent

weight off seat!

knees flexed, turned slightly inward

weight on balls of feet, slightly pigeon-toed

cranks level

No brakes *

With dynamic posture, your body acts as a giant shock absorbing system. This results in Ⓐ staying attached to the bike, and Ⓑ bouncing as a unit over fairly large obstacles at high speed. I always ride in this position offroad at high speeds so I'll be ready for unexpected trail anomalies. However, no matter how good you think you are, sometimes it is best to exercise good judgement and simply SLOW DOWN!

rider concentrating on the "event horizon" (ie - the immediate area of trail surface transition.

Event Horizon

*Pre-Crash Braking In most cases, forget about braking... sudden lock-up braking usually turns a marginal control situation into a no-control situation. A preemptory bunny-hop and good body/bike control is the ticket here...

Too late for brakes!!

hail mary....

rider concentrating on the end of the gnarly section

whew!

preemptive bunny-hop

ba-rump!

Shock is absorbed by wrists, arms, spine, knees, thighs, etc.

Riding Secrets Of
The
Totally Honed

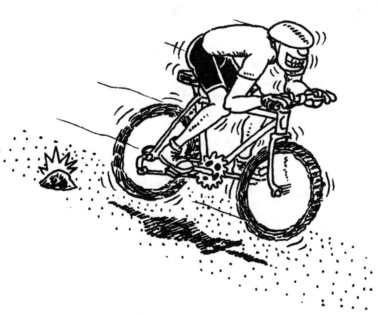

Riding Secrets Of The Totally Honed...

What follows is a collection of tips, tricks, arcane knowledge and strange advice (all of which was learned by repeatedly smashing into things...) that may provide a shortcut on the path to Mountain Bike Nirvana...

① G-forcing A Bunny Hop — You can cheat the complex body english required for a bunny hop by using a combination of high velocity & G-forces to launch the bike off a bump or hump or dip. Find a fast downhill with a potential launch pad, get going fast, compress your body before the hump (non-dynamically) and let the bump/hump/dip compress the tires... do the normal hop release at the peak and FLY!

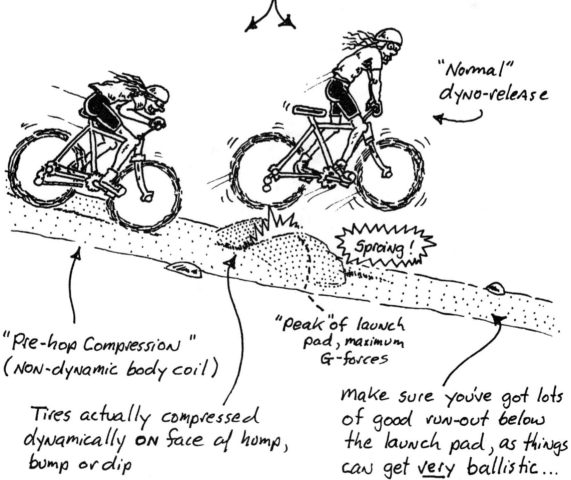

"Normal" dyno-release

Sproing!

"peak" of launch pad, maximum G-forces

"Pre-hop Compression" (non-dynamic body coil)

Tires actually compressed dynamically on face of hump, bump or dip

make sure you've got lots of good run-out below the launch pad, as things can get very ballistic...

② Not Swallowing A Bump - If you hit a bump at moderate to high speed standing with spine straight and arms & legs locked you will achieve a double launch... from the bump and from your bike! [See "Crash Wisdom".]

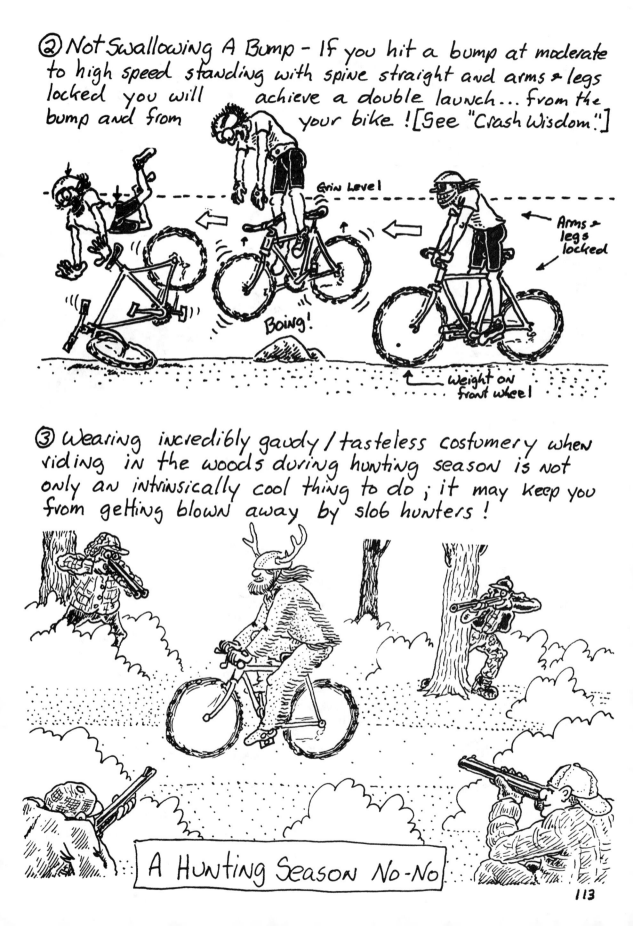

Grin Level

Boing!

Arms & legs locked

Weight on front wheel

③ Wearing incredibly gaudy/tasteless costumery when riding in the woods during hunting season is not only an intrinsically cool thing to do; it may keep you from getting blown away by slob hunters!

A Hunting Season No-No

④ How to tell if your buddy is seriously injured...

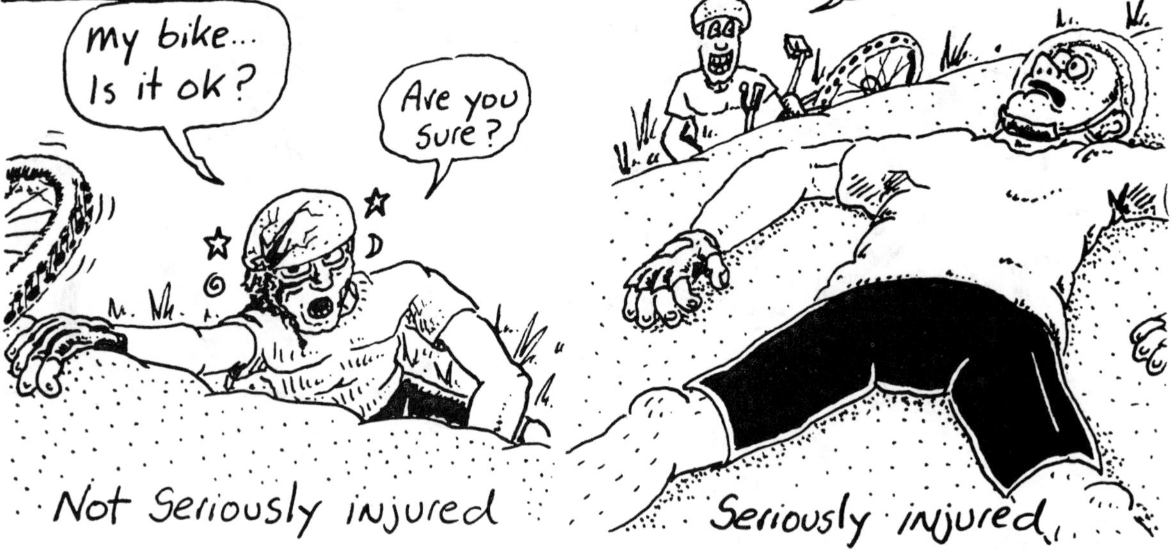

"my bike... Is it ok?"

"Are you sure?"

Not Seriously injured

"Your bike looks okay! Yo, Fred?"

"Fred?"

Seriously injured

⑤ Being a cool dude...

① Take frequent rest stops.
② Drink tons of water.
③ Go swimming or wading when possible.
④ Take micro-showers with your water bottle

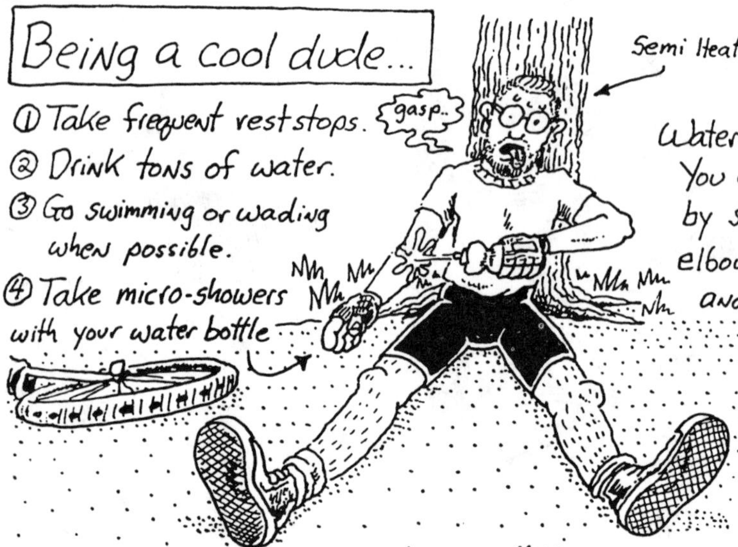

"gasp.."

Semi Heatstroke

Water Bottle Micro-Showers *
You can cool down quickly by squirting water on inner elbows, head, back of neck, and backs of knees....

Ahhhhh!

* If you've got water to spare! Water in your body is better than water on your body!

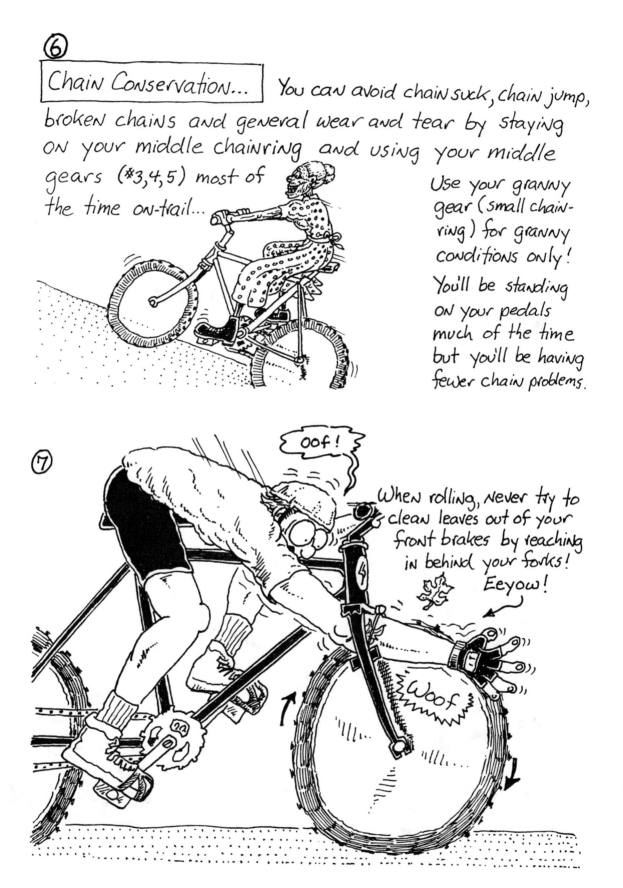

⑥

Chain Conservation... You can avoid chain suck, chain jump, broken chains and general wear and tear by staying on your middle chainring and using your middle gears (#3,4,5) most of the time on-trail...

Use your granny gear (small chainring) for granny conditions only!

You'll be standing on your pedals much of the time but you'll be having fewer chain problems.

⑦

oof!

When rolling, never try to clean leaves out of your front brakes by reaching in behind your forks! Eeyow!

Woof

115

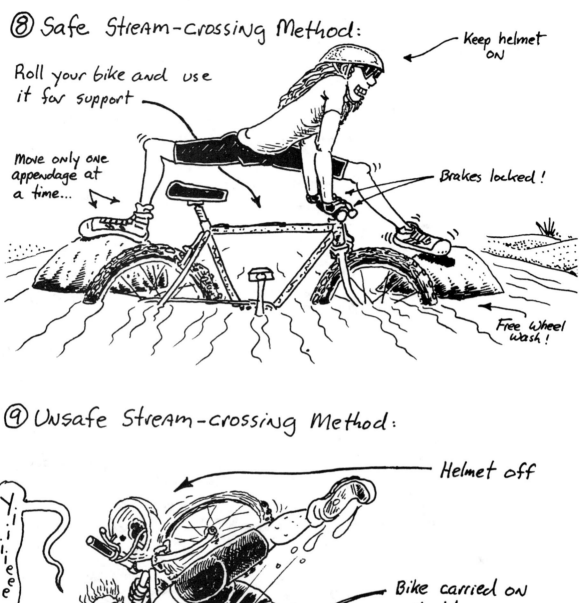

⑧ Safe Stream-crossing Method:

Roll your bike and use it for support

Keep helmet ON

Move only one appendage at a time...

Brakes locked!

Free Wheel Wash!

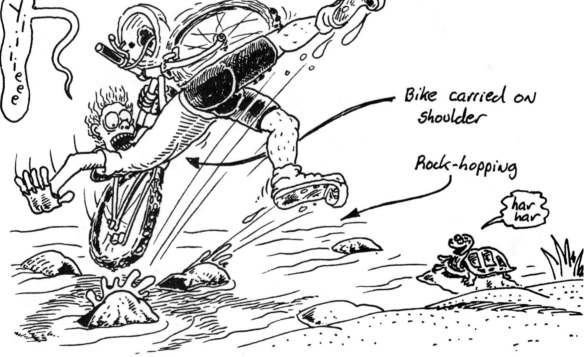

⑨ Unsafe Stream-crossing Method:

Yiiieee

Helmet off

Bike carried on shoulder

Rock-hopping

har har

⑩ And, speaking of streams...

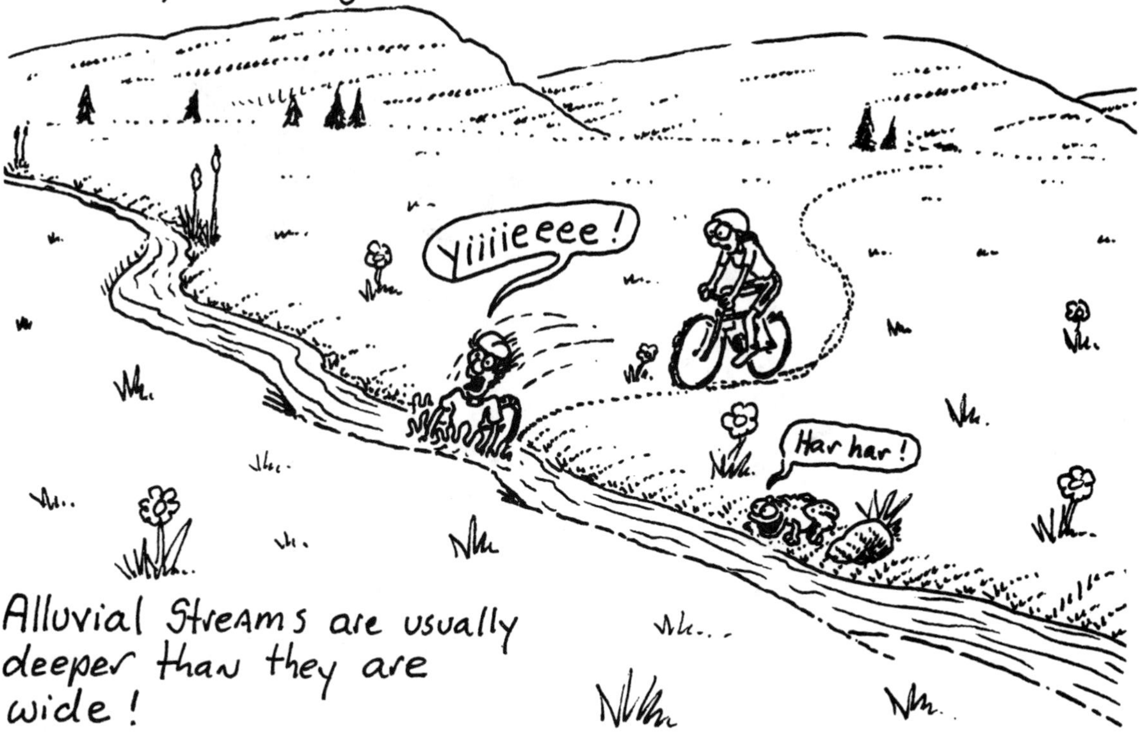

Yiiiieeee!

Har har!

Alluvial streams are usually deeper than they are wide!

⑪ Safe Quick-release Hub Lever Alignment

Always keep your quick-release hub levers positioned parallel to the ground and pointed rearward. This will prevent accidental snagging & releasing your hubs on trail. An accidental hub release while riding can be rather catastrophic to the rider...

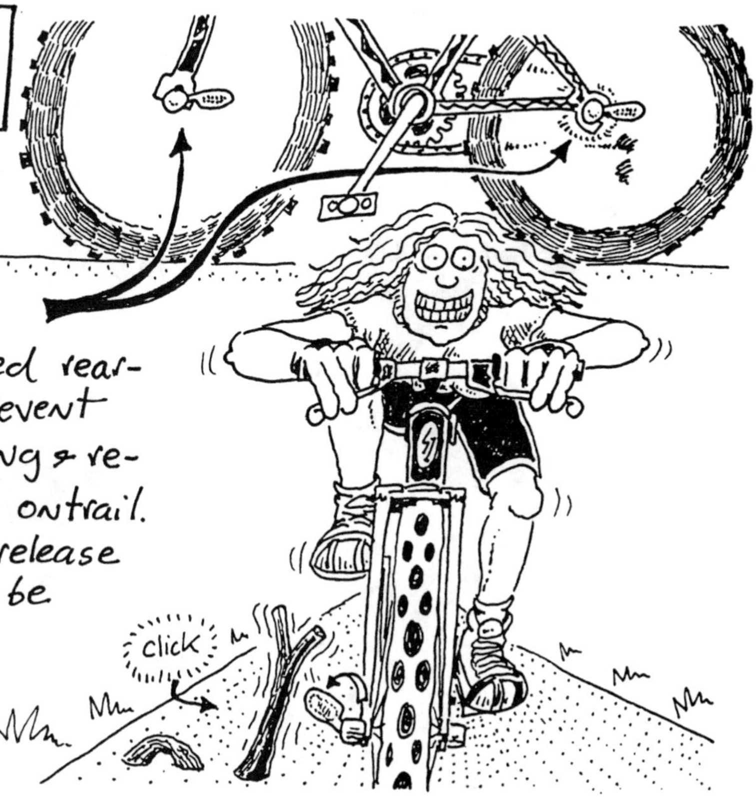

click

117

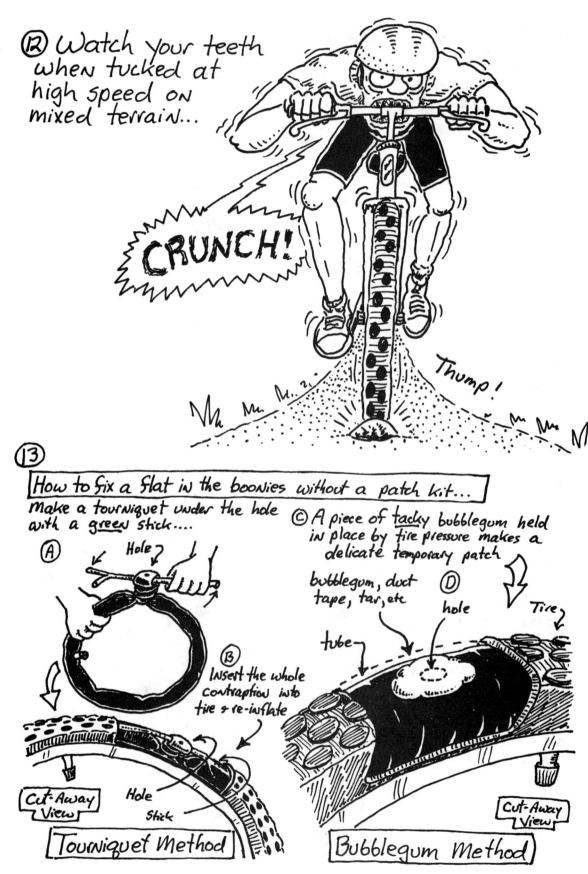

⑫ Watch your teeth when tucked at high speed on mixed terrain...

CRUNCH!

Thump!

⑬

How to fix a flat in the boonies without a patch kit...

make a tourniquet under the hole with a green stick....

Ⓐ

Hole

Ⓒ A piece of tacky bubblegum held in place by tire pressure makes a delicate temporary patch

bubblegum, duct tape, tar, etc

Ⓓ

hole

Tire

tube

Ⓑ Insert the whole contraption into tire & re-inflate

Cut-Away View

Hole

Stick

Tourniquet Method

Cut-Away View

Bubblegum Method

118

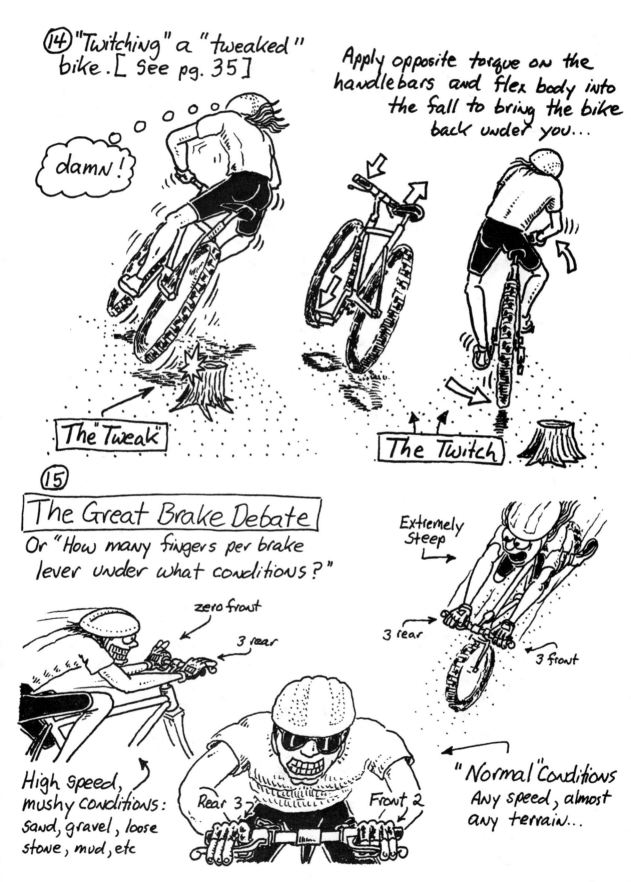

(14) "Twitching" a "tweaked" bike. [See pg. 35]

Apply opposite torque on the handlebars and flex body into the fall to bring the bike back under you...

damn!

The "Tweak"

The Twitch

(15)

The Great Brake Debate

Or "How many fingers per brake lever under what conditions?"

zero front

3 rear

Extremely Steep

3 rear

3 front

High speed, mushy conditions: sand, gravel, loose stone, mud, etc

Rear 3

Front 2

"Normal" Conditions Any speed, almost any terrain...

119

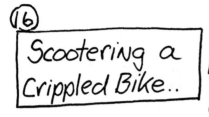

⑯ Scootering a Crippled Bike..

If you break a chain way back in the boonies (or pretzel a derailleur, etc.) and lack the proper tools for a road repair don't push your bike, scooter it!

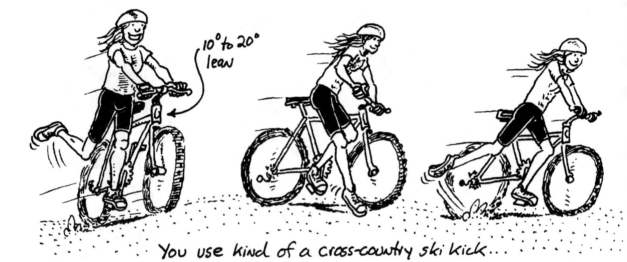

10° to 20° lean

You use kind of a cross-country ski kick...

17.) Advanced Scootering Technique... Looks awkward but gives the rider better balance: rider keeps correct foot on pedal and reaches around from behind with the other leg for the kick...

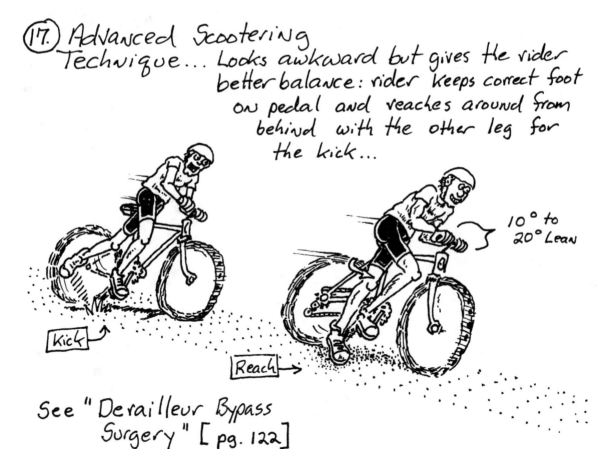

Kick

Reach →

10° to 20° Lean

See "Derailleur Bypass Surgery" [pg. 122]

⑱ How to weed out geeks at a glance....

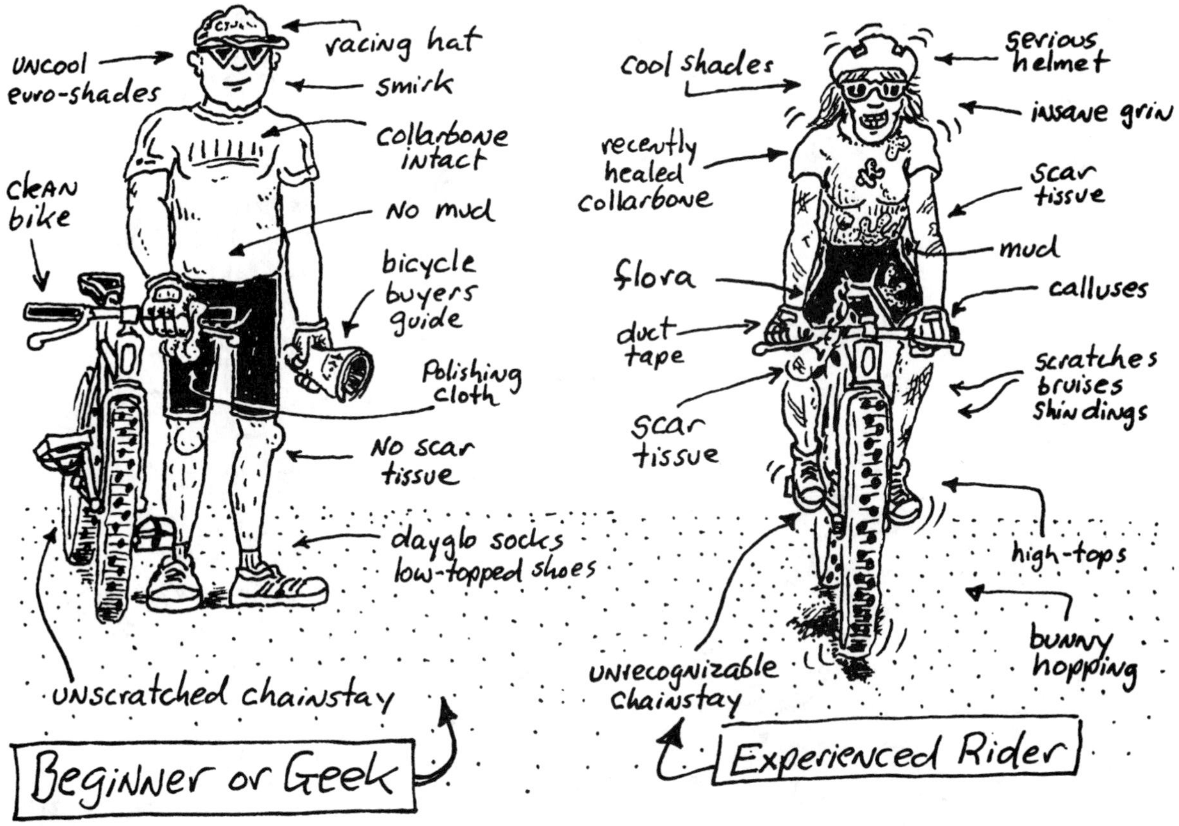

racing hat
UNcool euro-shades
smirk
collarbone intact
clean bike
No mud
bicycle buyers guide
Polishing cloth
No scar tissue
dayglo socks low-topped shoes
unscratched chainstay
Beginner or Geek
cool shades
serious helmet
insane grin
recently healed collarbone
scar tissue
mud
flora
calluses
duct tape
scratches bruises shin dings
scar tissue
high-tops
bunny hopping
unrecognizable chainstay
Experienced Rider

⑲ How To Tie Your Shoes

Getting a shoelace wrapped around the pedal axle or sucked into the chainwheel is always a nuisance and occasionally a disaster..

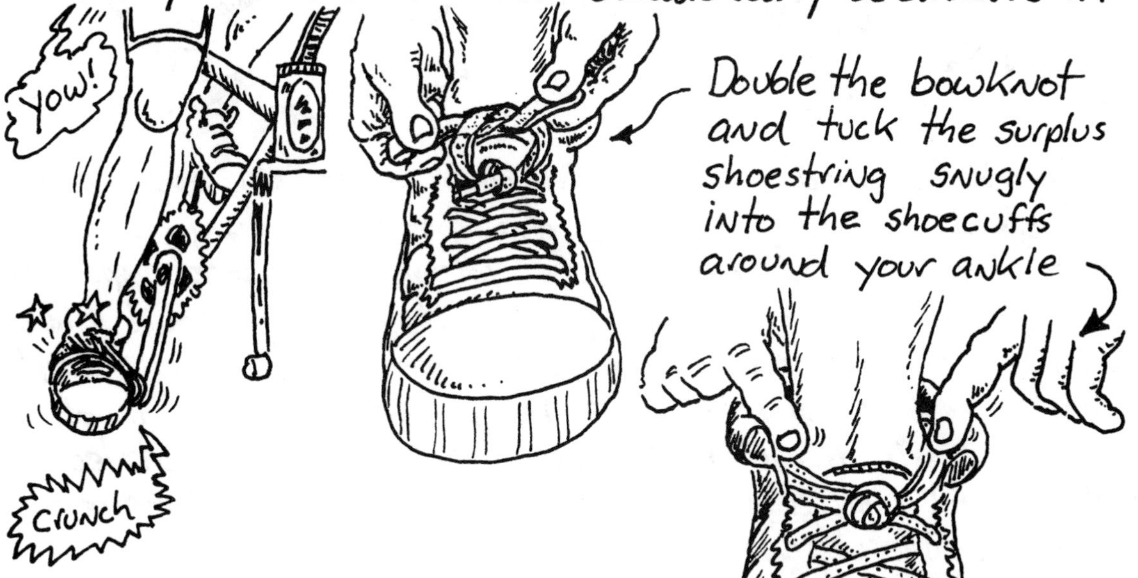

YOW!
CRUNCH
Double the bowknot and tuck the surplus shoestring snugly into the shoecuffs around your ankle

㉑ Derailleur Bypass Surgery — If you totally pretzel your derailleur way back in the boonies, don't despair. Simply whip out your 15 mm wrench and chaintool and take the derailleur out of the loop!

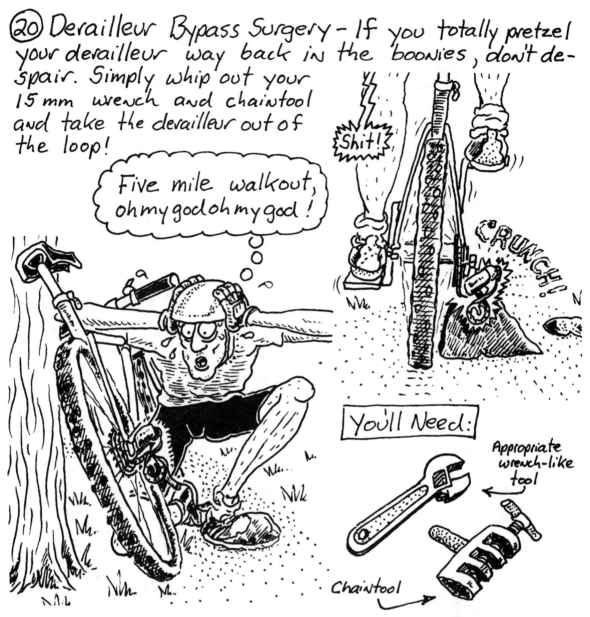

Five mile walkout, oh my god oh my god!

Shit!

CRUNCH!

You'll Need:

Appropriate wrench-like tool

Chaintool

① Break the chain, ② Remove derailleur, ③ Loosen wheel, ④ Select the most _suitable_ gear for pedalling out and set chain on that gear [Note: you may have to experiment a little with the next gear up or down for good wheel alignment with proper chain tension], ⑤ Remove surplus links and re-join the chain, ⑥ Realign wheel and check chain tension, ⑦ Pedal on out. Do not leave the dead derailleur lying on the trail... it'll make a great conversation piece and/or paperweight!

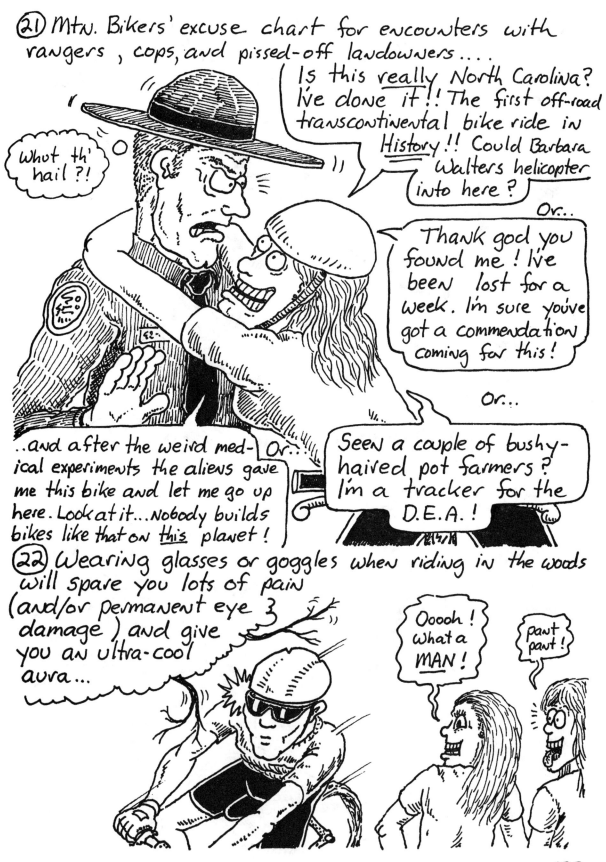

21 Mtn. Bikers' excuse chart for encounters with rangers, cops, and pissed-off landowners....

Whut th' hail?!

Is this really North Carolina? I've done it!! The first off-road transcontinental bike ride in History!! Could Barbara Walters helicopter into here?

Or...

Thank god you found me! I've been lost for a week. I'm sure you've got a commendation coming for this!

Or...

..and after the weird medical experiments the aliens gave me this bike and let me go up here. Look at it...Nobody builds bikes like that on this planet!

Or...

Seen a couple of bushy-haired pot farmers? I'm a tracker for the D.E.A.!

22 Wearing glasses or goggles when riding in the woods will spare you lots of pain (and/or permanent eye damage) and give you an ultra-cool aura...

Ooooh! What a MAN!

pant pant!

123

(23) Warning!! Gym shorts have a tendency to snag the nose of the seat in the crotch with unfortunate consequences when the rider goes to stand on the pedals...

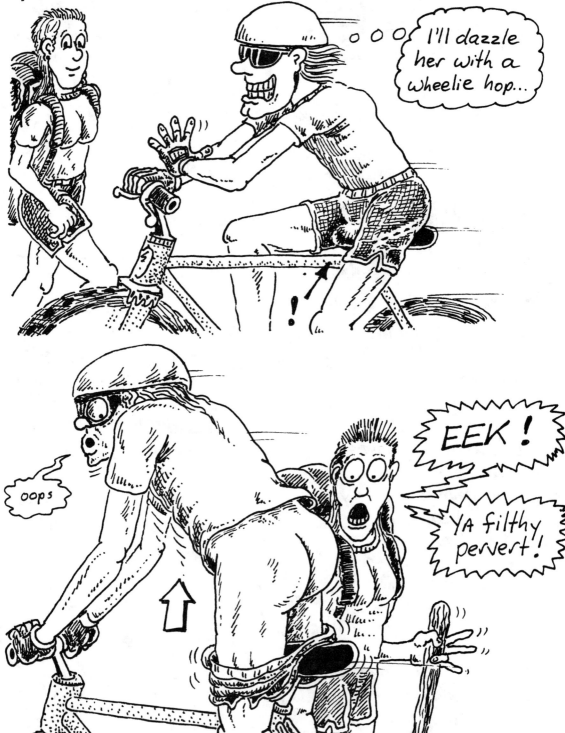

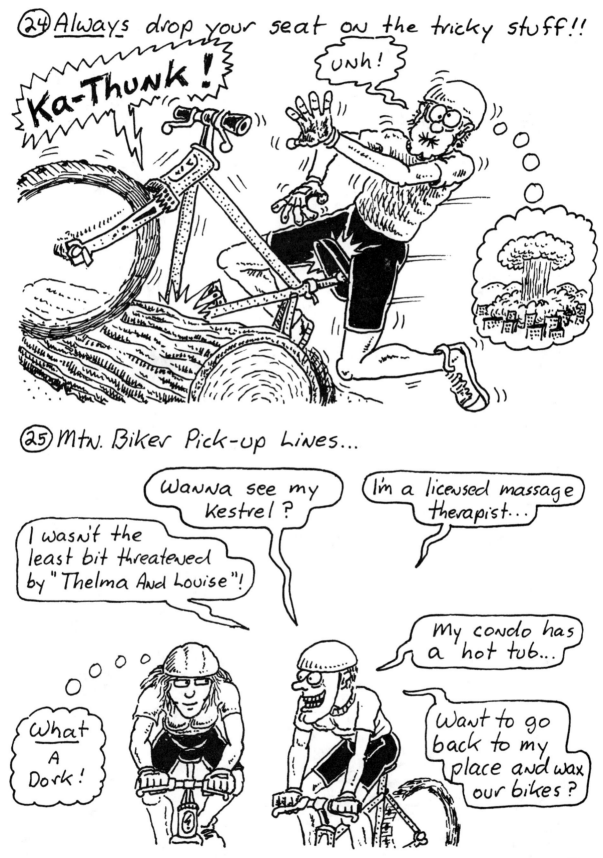

26) **Weight-shift Standing Climbing**[*] Here the rider shifts his/her weight from one leg to the other, using body weight to supercharge the normal pedal stroke. This weight-shifting imparts a side-to-side swinging motion to the bike which is contraindicated on an upgrade with a very

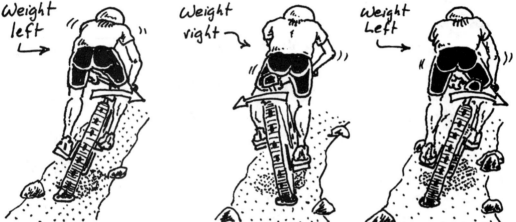

Weight left →

Weight right →

Weight left →

loose surface because the footprint of the tires changes on each swing. As a rule, when you're climbing a loose-surfaced upgrade you want to keep the bike as still as possible to maintain a constant "footprint."

[*A.K.A. "Honking"]

27) For persistant intermittent mechanical problems, bike exorcism may be necessary!

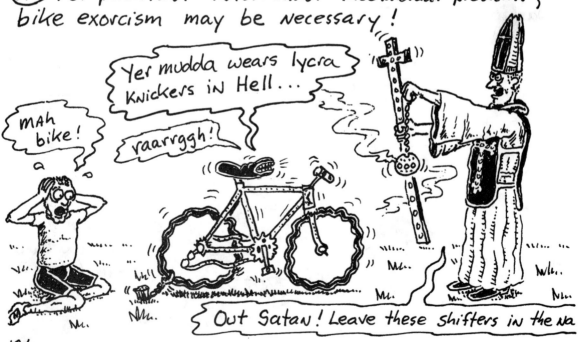

Yer mudda wears lycra knickers in Hell...

MAh bike!

raarrggh!

Out Satan! Leave these shifters in the Na

(28) Technoporn and Technoparanoia- "Technoparanoia" is the feeling of techno-inadequacy one gets from reading too many hyped-up product reviews in the various mtn. bike magazines (a.k.a. "technoporn"). While these pub-

pant pant

New ultimate Way Cool

Buyers Guide 1992

lications do occasionally disseminate useful in-formation, at best it's 80% hype. The best bike is the bike that fits you, not some new contraption a paid reviewer touts as the ultimate ride of the decade based on advertising revenue.

Gee...maybe my rims _are_ too narrow... the braking does feel a little too crisp... ...ohmygod, my bike's a DEATH-TRAP! ...I'll never be able to sell it... I got it! I'll give it to my girlfriend...

(29) Mtn. Bikers' Excuse Chart: (or "Why not to ride...")

Column A, environmental reasons:

"too hot"
"too cold"
"too wet"
"too dry"
"too early"
"too late"
"too long a ride"
"too short a ride"
"too hard a ride"
"too easy a ride"

Sorry, guys. It's (1) (I'm) Column A, B, or C

Column B, mechanical reasons
..."need to wax my bike"
..."need to adjust my shifters"
..."need to overhaul my derailleur."
..."need to repack my headset"

Column C, personal reasons:
"too busy", "too tired", "too bummed out over the plight of the Kurds," "thinking about trading in my bike" (see above), "fighting off a cold," etc.

So I won't be able to ride today...

Mtn. Bike Wax

(30) Dealing with non-human organic obstacles...

Tree Swiped (trē swīpd) v., To be struck a direct or glancing blow by a tree or trees in a vertical configuration (see "clothes-lined")

You can slalom thru spaces narrower than your handlebars by leaning the bike over and body thrusting thusly ①

Crunch!

② Trees can be contacted intentionally in truly desperate situations...

Troubleshooting Body Pain

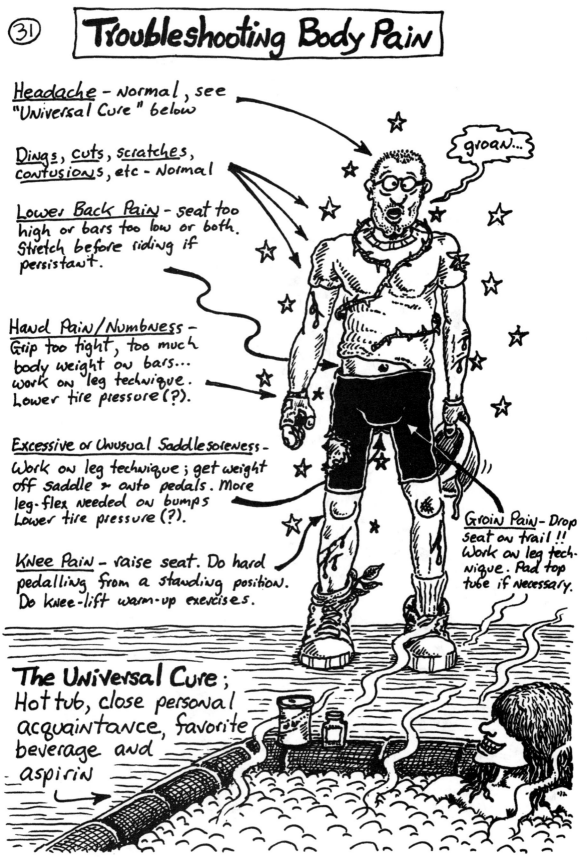

Headache - Normal, see "Universal Cure" below

Dings, cuts, scratches, contusions, etc - Normal

Lower Back Pain - seat too high or bars too low or both. Stretch before riding if persistant.

Hand Pain/Numbness - Grip too tight, too much body weight on bars... work on leg technique. Lower tire pressure (?).

Excessive or Unusual Saddle soreness - Work on leg technique; get weight off saddle & onto pedals. More leg-flex needed on bumps. Lower tire pressure (?).

Knee Pain - raise seat. Do hard pedalling from a standing position. Do knee-lift warm-up exercises.

groan...

Groin Pain - Drop seat on trail!! Work on leg technique. Pad top tube if necessary.

The Universal Cure; Hot tub, close personal acquaintance, favorite beverage and aspirin

32 How to keep ACCE$$ORIES fastened to your bike under rough (normal) conditions....

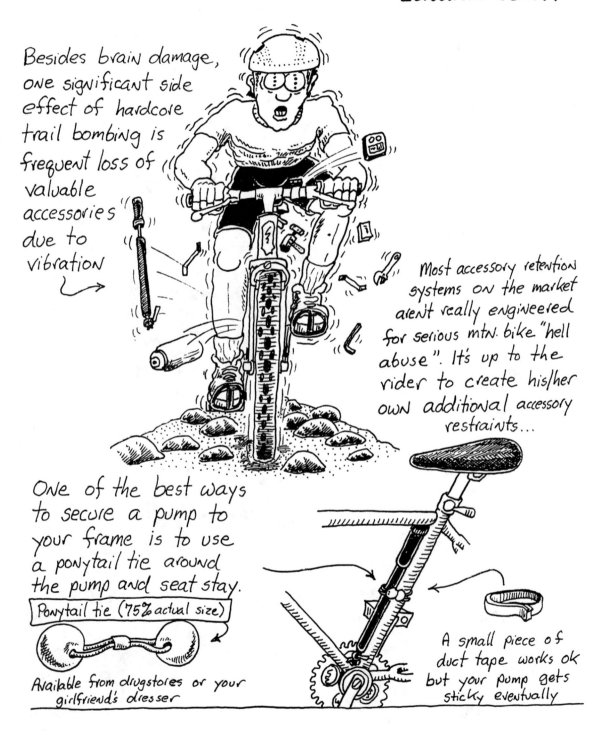

Besides brain damage, one significant side effect of hardcore trail bombing is frequent loss of valuable accessories due to vibration

Most accessory retention systems on the market aren't really engineered for serious mtn. bike "hell abuse". It's up to the rider to create his/her own additional accessory restraints...

One of the best ways to secure a pump to your frame is to use a ponytail tie around the pump and seat stay.

Ponytail tie (75% actual size)

Available from drugstores or your girlfriend's dresser

A small piece of duct tape works ok but your pump gets sticky eventually

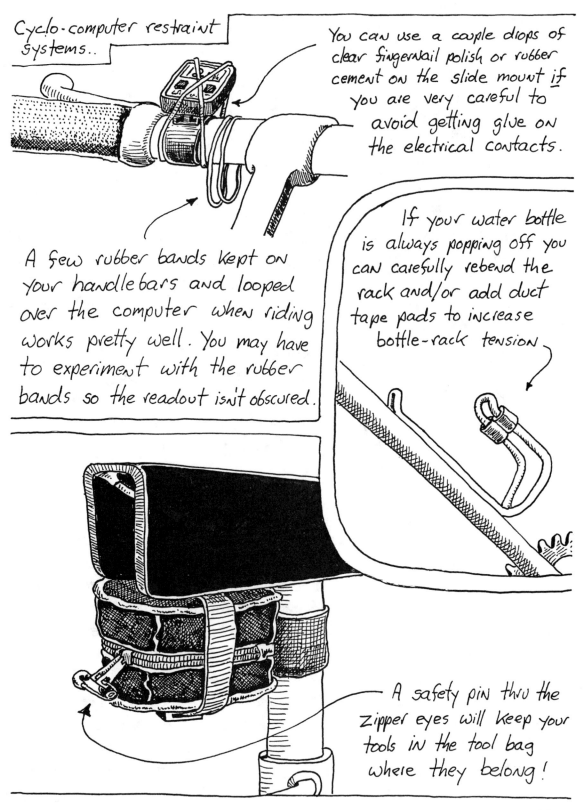

Cyclo-computer restraint systems..

You can use a couple drops of clear fingernail polish or rubber cement on the slide mount if you are very careful to avoid getting glue on the electrical contacts.

A few rubber bands kept on your handlebars and looped over the computer when riding works pretty well. You may have to experiment with the rubber bands so the readout isn't obscured.

If your water bottle is always popping off you can carefully rebend the rack and/or add duct tape pads to increase bottle-rack tension

A safety pin thru the zipper eyes will keep your tools in the tool bag where they belong!

33) Ride A Well-Tuned Bike!

Unless you are a qualified bike mechanic, periodically take your bike to your friendly neighborhood bike shop for a "tune up".*Observe the mechanic so you can learn to do it yourself eventually. If management won't let you hang out in the shop with the gearhead working on your bike, find a new bike shop!
*Tune Up - Close inspection and general tightening up of the entire bike by a qualified mechanic.

34) Establishing a "safe" trail speed-

"Safe" trail speed is subject to a lot of variables (surface, presence or absence of organic & inorganic obstacles, etc.) but under most conditions the "Event Horizon" sets your speed. Event Horizon can be defined as either "maximum sight distance" or "minimum distance to a peak move". Whichever applies, the rider should maintain a speed that will allow him/her to stop or slow down sufficiently to deal with whatever pops up on his/her event horizon. On the opposite page (top) the rider is cruising too fast relative to his event horizon. He hasn't allowed sufficient time to react to trail variables. As speed increases, distance to the event horizon decreases! ↗

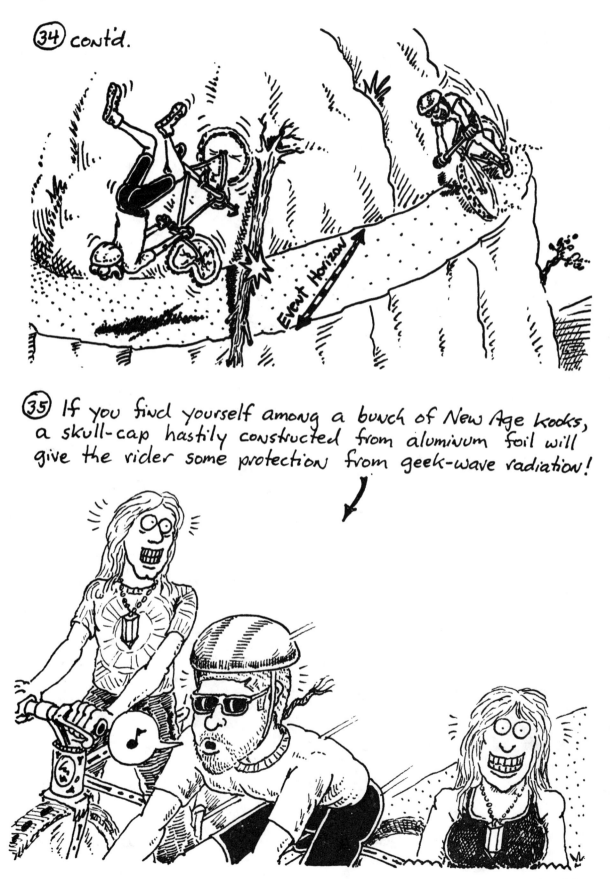

Event Horizon

(35) If you find yourself among a bunch of New Age kooks, a skull-cap hastily constructed from aluminum foil will give the rider some protection from geek-wave radiation!

36) You can keep your sneakers dry by ratcheting across/thru shallow creeks and/or puddles...

37) Metaphorical "Mountain Music"... the mountain is the record*, you're the stylus...

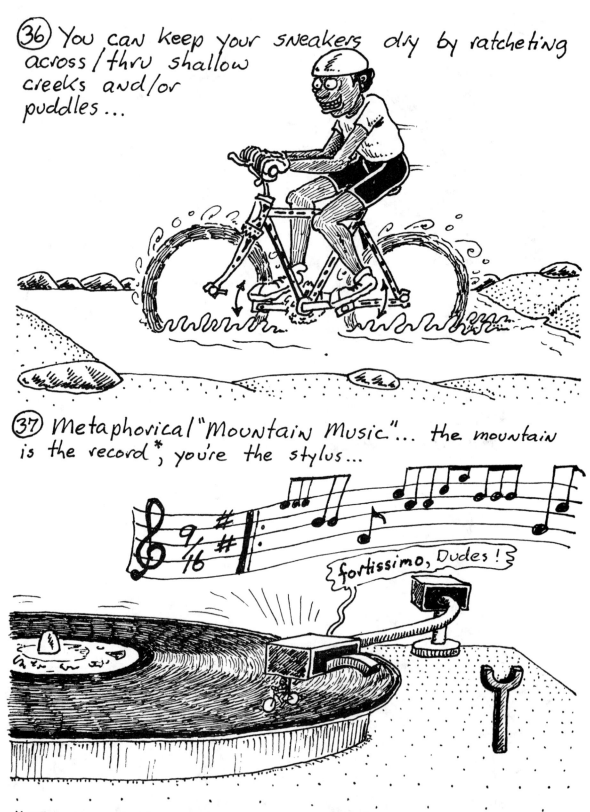

* This is probably meaningful only to those of us who are old enough to know what an actual "record" *is*!

(38) This hasn't got diddly to do with advanced riding technique but I'm desperate... Would somebody please build a mountain bike with the derailleur in a less vulnerable spot?! If you think about it, they couldn't have picked a worse spot to put it, dangling way down there under the freewheel. Anyhow, I thought about it some over a few beers and came up with this —

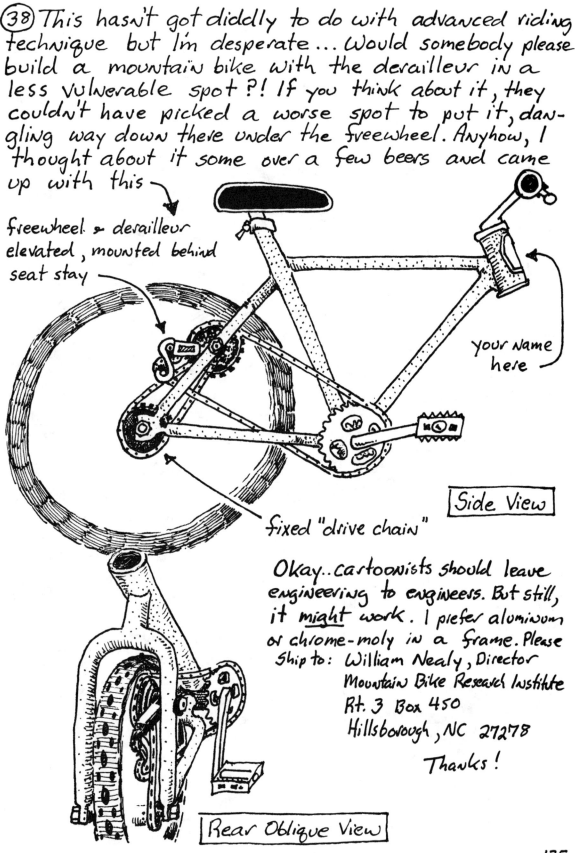

freewheel & derailleur elevated, mounted behind seat stay

your name here

fixed "drive chain"

Side View

Okay.. cartoonists should leave engineering to engineers. But still, it _might_ work. I prefer aluminum or chrome-moly in a frame. Please ship to: William Nealy, Director Mountain Bike Research Institute Rt. 3 Box 450 Hillsborough, NC 27278

Thanks!

Rear Oblique View

39 Toe Clip Or Not Toe Clip
(or "Why We Wear Chinese Toe Cuffs...")

Toe clip or not toe clip, that is the question. Whether 'tis nobler in the mind to suffer the dings and contusions of unclipp'd riding, or to bind thy feet against a sea of gnarly singletrack and by these contraptions, ride o'er them with ease. To clip.. to slip no more, and by clipping to end the buttache and the thousand natural shocks that feet are heir to; 'tis a consummation devoutly to be honed. No clip, to slip — to slip perchance to be trashed most heinously. Ay, there's the rub...

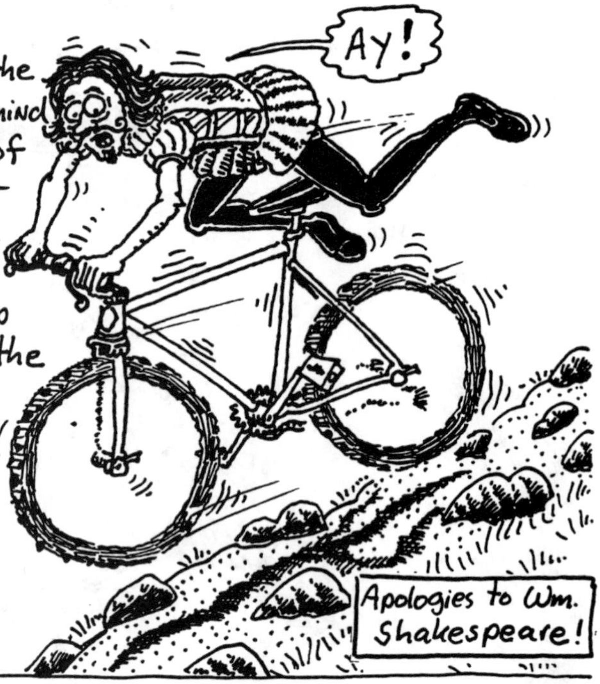

AY!

Apologies to Wm. Shakespeare!

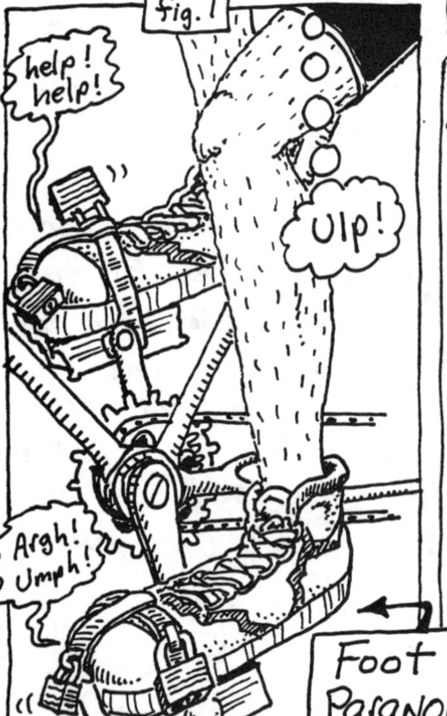

fig. 1

help! help!

Ulp!

Argh! Umph!

Foot Paranoia

Learning to wear toe clips on the trail is a major mountain bike rite of passage, usually marking the transition from intermediate to advanced riding. Most people find toe clips (a.k.a. "toe cuffs") to be very claustrophobic initially (see fig. 1). This is probably because most riders get in the habit of catching falls by sliding their feet laterally off the pedals. A foot will <u>not</u> come out of a toe clip sideways! The best toe clip escape move is to relax your toes and push straight down on the back of the pedal — the pedal literally rolls off the foot (fig 2).

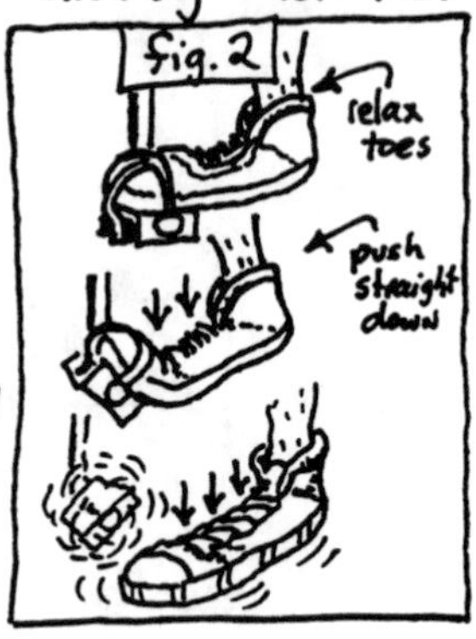

fig. 2

relax toes

push straight down

The main advantage of toe clipping on trails is a very secure stance which gives you a platform for some serious body english. You'll also have more power and no matter how bumpy the trail gets, your feet will stay on the pedals! Start on easy trails with the straps loose and slowly work your way up to hard trails and snug (not tight!) straps. Your feet will get habituated to the clips in the process. Use trees, etc. for stability when getting into toe clips initially (fig. 3). On smooth stretches practice rolling the pedals and inserting toes on the fly.

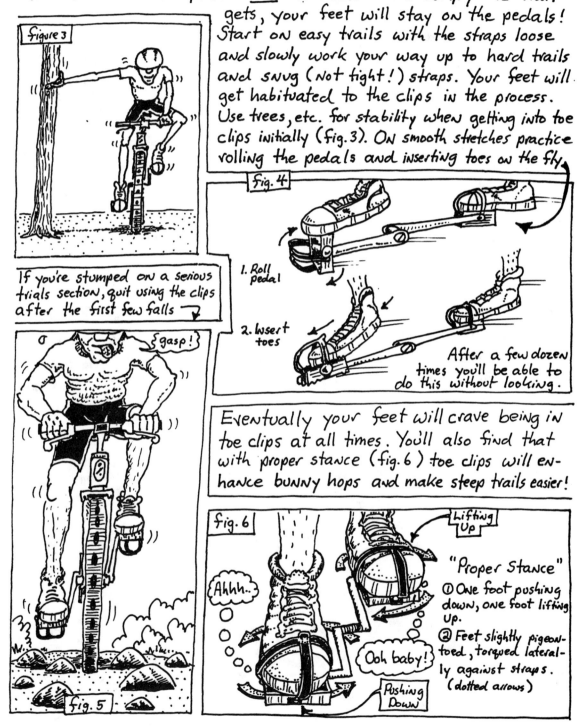

figure 3

If you're stumped on a serious trials section, quit using the clips after the first few falls ⟶

fig. 4

1. Roll pedal

2. Insert toes

After a few dozen times you'll be able to do this without looking.

gasp!

fig. 5

Eventually your feet will crave being in toe clips at all times. You'll also find that with proper stance (fig. 6) toe clips will enhance bunny hops and make steep trails easier!

fig. 6

Lifting Up

Ahhh..

Ooh baby!

Pushing Down

"Proper Stance"
① One foot pushing down, one foot lifting up.
② Feet slightly pigeon-toed, torqued laterally against straps. (dotted arrows)

(40) All about seat height...

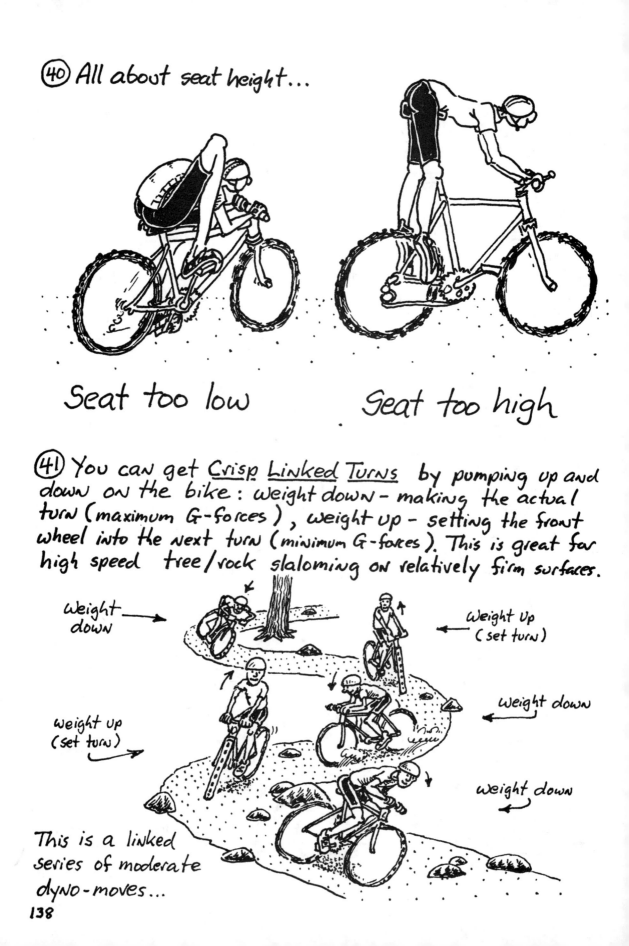

Seat too low   Seat too high

(41) You can get <u>Crisp</u> <u>Linked</u> <u>Turns</u> by pumping up and down on the bike: weight down - making the actual turn (maximum G-forces), weight up - setting the front wheel into the next turn (minimum G-forces). This is great for high speed tree/rock slaloming on relatively firm surfaces.

Weight down →

Weight Up
(set turn) ←

weight down ←

weight up
(set turn) ↘

weight down ↙

This is a linked series of moderate dyno-moves...

Philosophy, Ethics, Survival and some Stupid Bike Tricks...

Mtn. Bike Ethics

Ethical Guideline #1 - Protect and preserve the mountain bike environment... RIDE GENTLY! Ride in designated areas only... repair all trail damage you encounter or cause... use dynamic riding techniques only under appropriate trail conditions... avoid wet weather trail riding ...etc. In short, take care of the trail environment and it will take care of you.

Ethical Guideline #2 - Ride Courteously! Avoid spooking or alienating hikers, horses, wildlife and other organic obstacles. If you want to ride like a maniac (we all do!) find an appropriate area to do so, away from the geeks! When you ride, consider yourself the Supreme Ambassador Of The Mountain Bike Nation! Pressure to exclude mtn. bikes from the woods is not going away anytime soon. Every time a mtn. biker rides like a slob we all pay the price. I say shoot 'em or make them be road cyclists!

Ethical Guideline #3 - Take responsibility for your riding actions! Repair trails, be courteous, rescue yourself, and, for god's sake, don't sue anybody! Every time some pinhead sues a landowner, outfitter, equipment manufacturer, bike shop, etc. this sport dies a little. Face it, this is a dangerous activity taking place in a potentially dangerous physical environment so people are going to get hurt. It's normal!

Obviously a faultily manufactured cantilever arm... I'm gonna sue!

Yiiieee!

Thunk

The Philosophical Precepts Of Modern Mountain Biking...

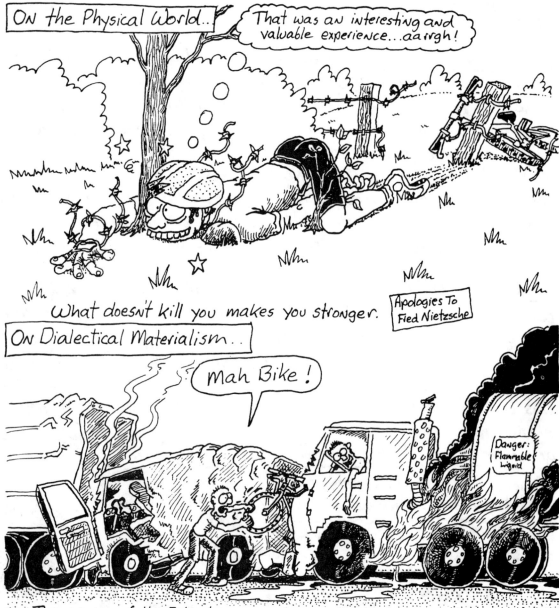

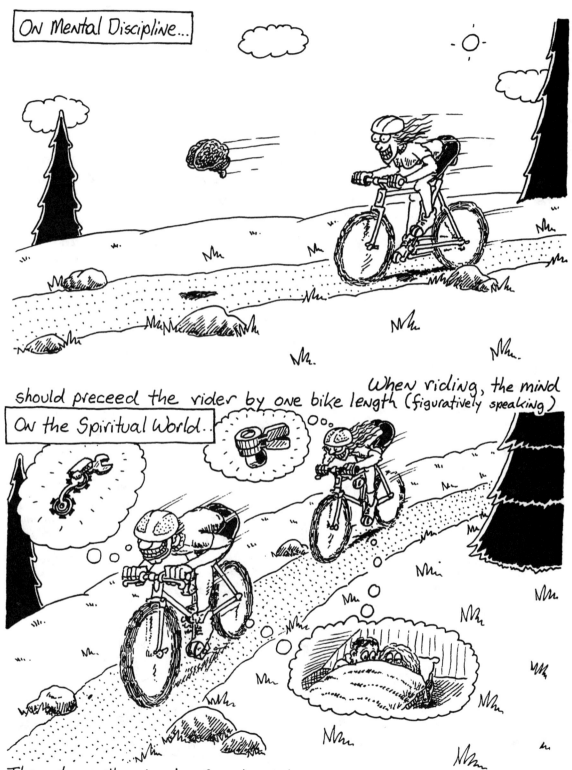

On Mental Discipline...

When riding, the mind should preceed the rider by one bike length (figuratively speaking)

On the Spiritual World.

The only worthy objects of contemplation are new components and sex...

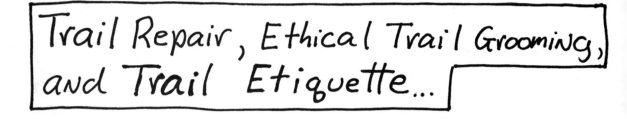

Trail Repair, Ethical Trail Grooming, and Trail Etiquette...

All trail users (hikers, bikers, & equestrians) have a negative impact on the trails they use. Being highly visible and controversial, mountain bikers have a special responsibility to protect and maintain the trails they use. The easiest form of trail maintenance is **Damage Prevention**; Always avoid skids, ride gently and carry wet sections! You can easily carry the following trail repair tools when you ride: folding pruning saw, garden trowel, and/or entrenching tool. Don't forget a pair of workgloves too!

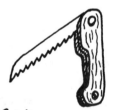
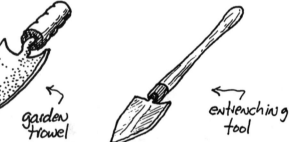

folding pruning saw

garden trowel

entrenching tool

A common form of mountain bike-related trail damage is the downhill-skid-on-steep-trail-rut-becomes-gully syndrome.

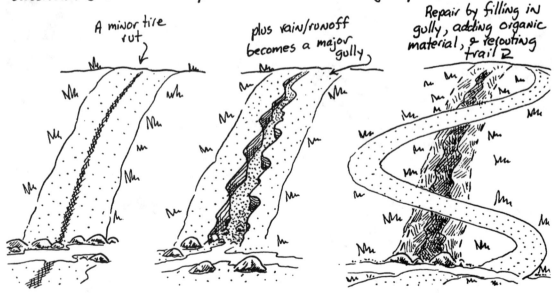

A minor tire rut

plus rain/runoff becomes a major gully

Repair by filling in gully, adding organic material, & rerouting trail ⤵

Runoff flowing down the fall-line of a trail causes severe erosion. You can create "water bars" to divert water laterally off the trail by ① digging a trench, ② building a berm, or ③ stepping with logs or rocks

Consider rerouting steep trail sections that require constant maintenance...

Flow

Berm

Step

Flow

Flow

Trench

Another mountain bike-vulnerable trail feature is the boggy trail segment. Eventually this will become a bottomless hog wallow. You can make such sections rideable by draining the trail and laying crosswise sticks to prevent tires from sinking into the muck. If you can't drain it, reroute the trail or carry the boggy part.

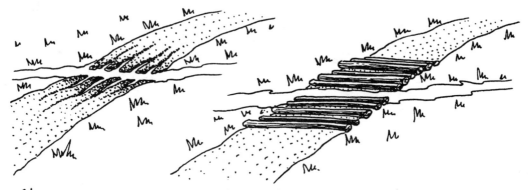

Always get permission from the landowner/land manager before conducting major trail repairs!

Ethical Trail Grooming

Justification #1 - The detour around the fallen tree will damage mosses & ferns as well as cause erosion on the high side of the trail.

To cut or NOT to cut..

Just in case a fut[ure] biker wants to ju[mp] it, I'll make my c[ut] small & to the sid[e] (dotted line)

Justification #2 - The tree is so high above the trail NO mortal mtn bikest can jump it. [Expert trials riders excepted]

Justification #3 - A detour on the low side is NOT feasible.

Unethical Trail Grooming

Indictment #1 - Chain tooth marks indicate the log was "in play" for a number of cyclists

Indictment #2 - Knowing the log was "in play", the cut could have been made to either side instead of smack in the middle, 16" wide instead of 4'.

Whew!

Can't wait to try "THE Log"!

A NON-permanent log climb overpass can be constructed with rocks & deadwood in minutes →

Indictment #3 - A detour was already well-established and caused little erosion.

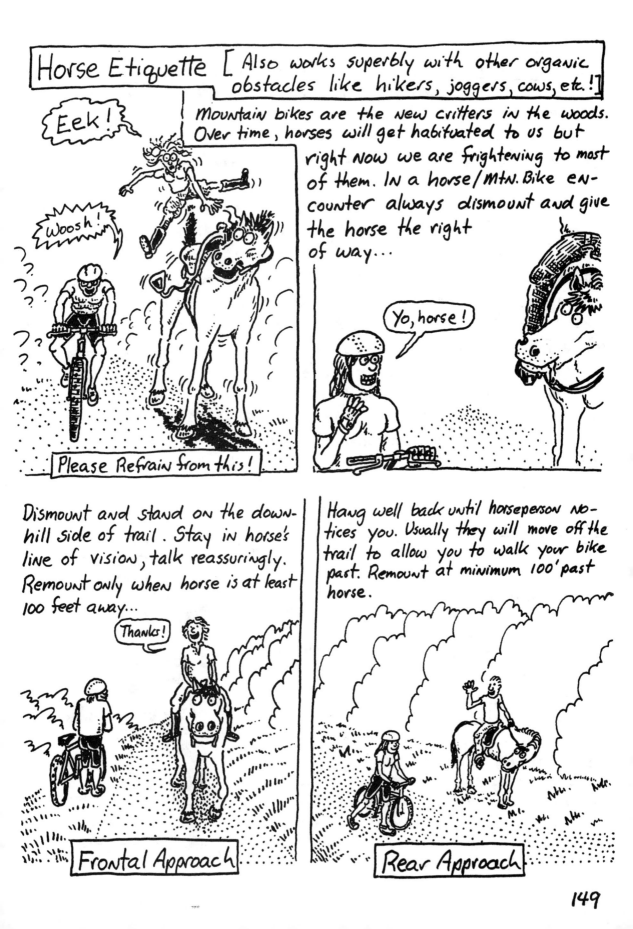

149

Survival Intro

Anyone who choses to recreate in the woods has a basic responsibility to themselves & their riding partners to learn a few simple wilderness survival skills. The information is abundant and usually free if you take the trouble to find it...

① "Orientating" - knowing where you are: the lie of the land, which way is North, which way is out, etc. [This is a simpler skill than "Orienteering" which deals with directions as a virtual science!] Good "orientating" keeps you from getting lost and facilitates self-rescue if you do.

② Emergency First Aid - Free courses, American Red Cross

③ Emergency Bike Repair - Hang out with gear-heads and learn how to keep your bike rolling with chewing gum, duct tape and wire. Free!

④ Self Rescue - How to get un-lost, how to set up an emergency shelter, build a fire, find water, food, etc. Try the public library.

.Your brain is your most important piece of survival equipment! Even if you have spare parts, bivy bags, Rambo knives, compasses, flares, radios, etc., if you're making bad decisions you are still basically screwed. Please take the time to learn these skills before you need them!

Dress For Success!

Probably the most important aspect of dressing for a cold weather mtn. bike ride is not wearing too much! [see opposite, top]. If it's a ride into a remote and unfamiliar location the wise mtn. biker will plan for all contingencies by carrying additional clothing such as wind pants, sweater, wool socks, wool hat, and an emergency bivi kit [see next page]. Because of weather variables it's best to have a pretty versatile layering system available to make necessary thermal adjustments.

helmet liner
goggles
Neck gaiter
polypro, pile, etc
wind shell
ski gloves
extra clothes
polypro, etc
wool socks

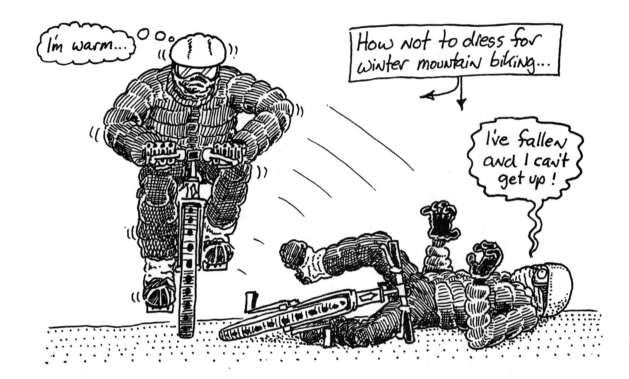

Backcountry Emergency Bivi Kit

If you get lost or hurt in the boonies in inclement weather this can save your life and the whole package weighs 8 ounces. Note: obviously we're talking about an extreme situation here. Unless you are hurt, hypothermic, and/or hopelessly lost it is usually best to keep moving if at all possible.

Emergency Bivi Kit Contents:
2 mylar survival "blankets"
1 box waterproof matches
1 candle
1 small aluminum teapot (to make hot beverages)
teabags, powdered drink mix (optional)
food (optional)

Survival Shelter: In a sheltered spot make a big pile of dry organic material (leaves, moss). Cover with one blanket. Wrap up in the other blanket, crawl into the middle of the pile and snuggle!

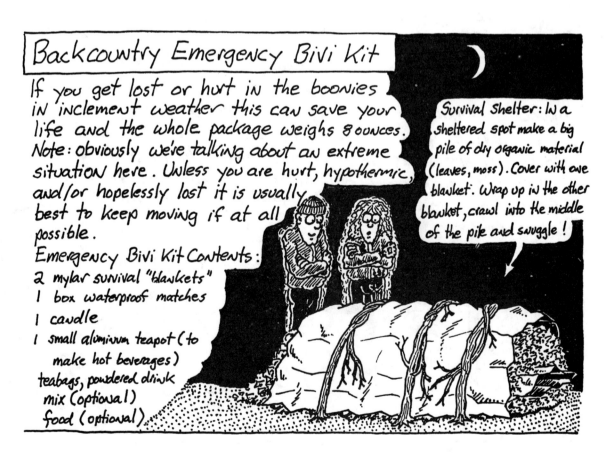

Lost In Space...

gasp!

I'm gonna kill you and your "shortcut"

Hey, we're not lost, we're in Western North Carolina! Yo, anybody got any water left?

"Demi-lost" (see below)

If you spend a lot of time riding in the boonies you're gonna get lost occasionally. There are two basic varieties of "lost"— Demi-lost and Mega-lost. Demi-lost is a state of being slightly confused within a known section of terrain (see above). Mega-lost is being totally disoriented in an essentially unknown (to you) section of terrain. If you follow a few basic Anti-lost protocols you can effectively innoculate yourself from ever becoming profoundly Mega-lost:

1. Familiarize yourself with the general area you'll be riding in. If there isn't a map available to take with you, look at a map and try to form a mental picture of the general area with self-rescue in mind...

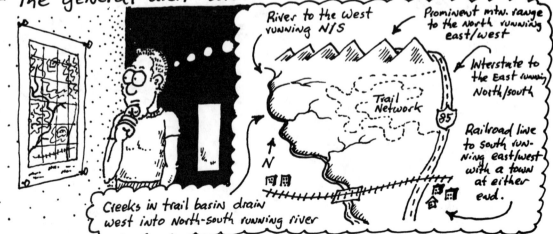

River to the West running N/S

Prominent mtn. range to the North running east/west

Interstate to the East running North/south

Trail Network

85

Railroad line to south running east/west with a town at either end.

N

Creeks in trail basin drain west into North-south running river

② Always know which way is North (use compass if necessary)!

③ Occasionally stop and look back uptrail for landmarks in case you have to retrace your route in.

④ Never _ever_ bushwhack blind!! Leave a trail only as a last resort _and_ with a specific goal in sight or within earshot (highway sounds, power lines, distant buildings, etc.). Remember, you can never be truly mega-lost standing on a trail! If you leave a trail, always mark your way so that you can _easily_ return to the trail if necessary.

⑤ Manage your time! If you're exploring an unfamiliar area keep in mind; "In-time equals out-time _sometimes_!" For example, if you've ridden a couple hours downhill into some mystery terrain, you'll need to allow a sizeable chunk of time _plus_ the original _time-in_ to compensate for a long uphill return! ⑥ Be prepared to bivy when riding in remote areas. An injury, breakdown or short period of demi-lostdom can put you in a life-threatening situation. Carrying matches, food, water, extra clothing and shelter-makings can save your life! [See p. 151]

⑦ Never move from relative strength to relative weakness in an emergency situation. If it's nearly dark and your party is mega-lost, tired, and semi-chilled STOP NOW! Stay on the trail, set up a shelter, build a fire and conserve your strength. True, there are times when it's advisable to push on in a bad situation (like if you're 2 miles from your truck and it's snowing). However, if you are truly mega-lost, pushing on in deteriorating conditions can kill you!

⑧ Don't panic! Unless you're a total pinhead you'll survive. Think of your situation as a great learning opportunity![1]

⑨ Always tell a responsible person *where you're going & when you expect to be back. The only thing worse than being mega-lost is being forgotten and mega-lost...

⑩ Seek out good instruction in wilderness survival, first aid, and emergency bike repair _before_ you put yourself in a wilderness survival situation.

*_Not_ the guys at the bar the night before!

[1] See "Philosophical Precept" #1 pg 144

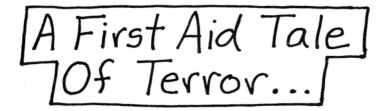

A First Aid Tale Of Terror...

Once upon a time in western North Carolina a group of highly experienced outdoorspeople were having a collective religious experience on some exceptional horse trails in a remote area when suddenly...

Eeeeeeyaaaaah!

damn!

Thud

Screeech!

Two of the bikers were EMT's trained in wilderness emergencies...

I'll get the first aid kit!

I'd call that an anterior dislocation.

What a lump! You want to try to reduce it? It's a long way out...

Your bike looks OK.

Aaaaaarrrrrghhhh...

my bike! my bike!

They placed their friend on a deadfall with a dangling weight to place gentle traction on the shoulder and, hopefully, pop it back in the socket...

gasp... groan aaarrrgh!

damn!

*Kids, don't try this at home !!!

The "Man Called Horse" method* of dislocation reduction is controversial but it often works.

45 minutes later...

Hey! You know what.. this is a broken collarbone, not a dislocation!

whoops!

That explains the lump!

whoops!

whoops!

Sorry, dude... really sorry...

malpractice malpractice malpractice..

He survived the first aid* and the collarbone healed up just fine. whew!

*A.K.A. "Chi-Chi"

While advanced first aid training is a must for backcountry mtn. bikers, mountain bike medics should always be mindful of the most important rule of emergency medicine..."Do No harm".

And finally...
Stupid Bike Tricks!

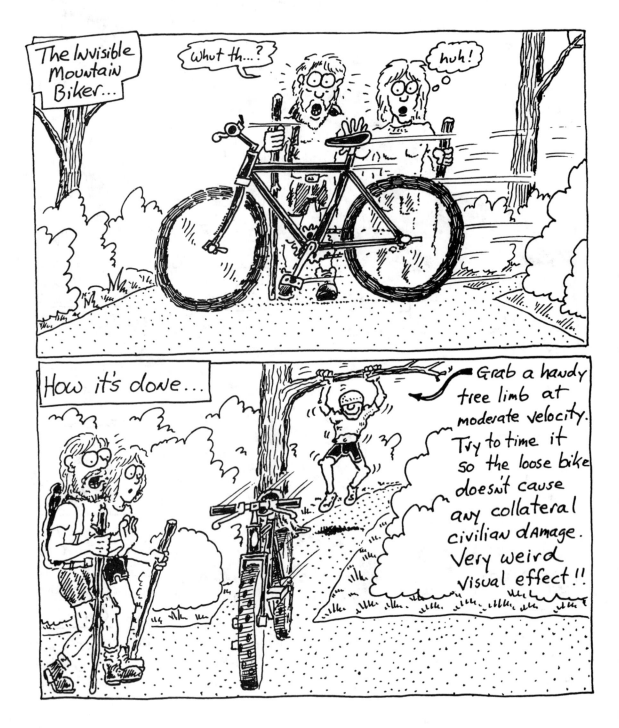

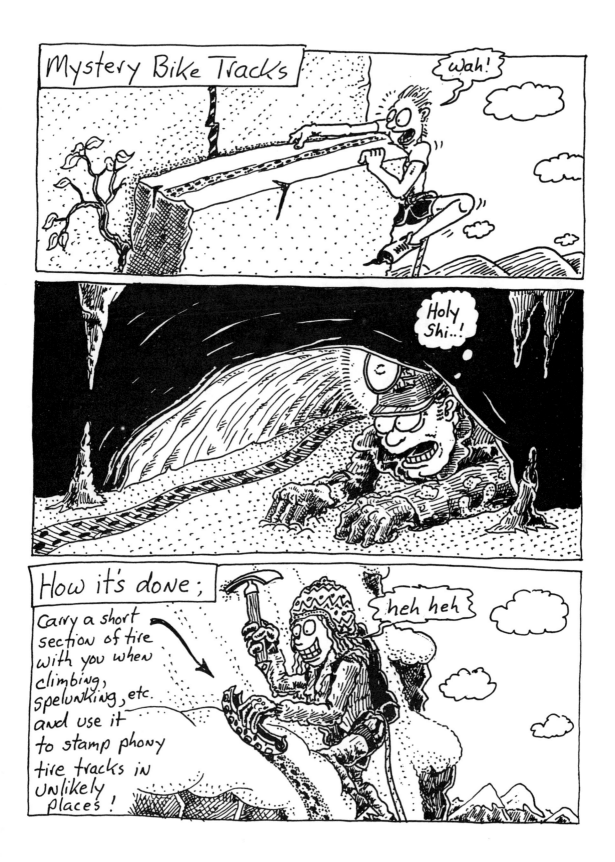

Bikespeak
[Selected Glossary]

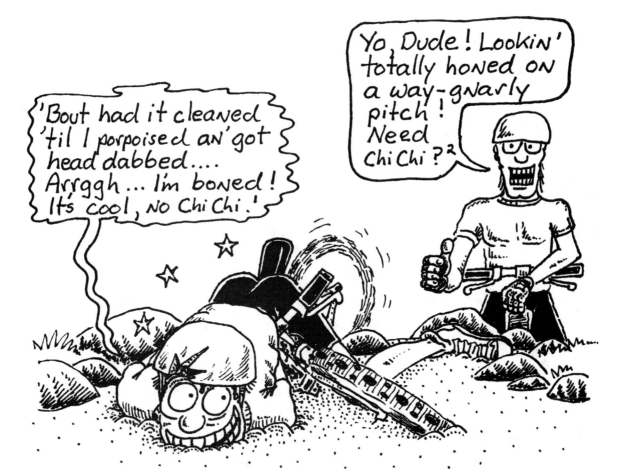

'Bout had it cleaned 'til I porpoised an' got head dabbed.... Arrggh... I'm boned! It's cool, No ChiChi.'

Yo, Dude! Lookin' totally honed on a way-gnarly pitch! Need ChiChi?[2]

[1]Trans: "I nearly made it without putting my foot down but I lost control and landed on my face.. Ouch! There is a seat in my rectum! First aid won't be necessary.

[2]Trans: "Hey, friend! You were looking very graceful on this highly technical section of trail. Do you need first aid?"

159

Bike speak...

__aerobic__ - muscle activity fuelled by inspired oxygen.

__anaerobic__ - intense muscle activity with energy provided without utilization of inspired oxygen. This is strenuous exercise confined to short bursts of activity. See "blown","legburn","micro-rest"

__blown__ - to lose peak muscle function (usually) after extended anaerobic exercise. Also, to exceed the credit limit on your charge card, as in; "Sorry sir, your Visa card is blown"...

__bomb__ - to descend a section of trail at an extremely high velocity.

__boned__ - to dynamically catch the nose of your seat in the posterior portion of your anatomy. See "groin plant"

__bunny hop__ - to pop the bike off the ground by compressing both wheels and bouncing in a pogo-like manner. Both wheels leave the ground simultaneously! See "Wheelie Hop".

__caterpillaring__ - jerky pedal cadence fluctuating between very fast and very slow. Extremely inefficient pedalling!

__Chi Chi (chēē chēē)__ first aid or first aid proceedure.

__clean__ - to ride a difficult trail section without dabbing.

__clothes lined__ - knocked off your bike by a suspended obstacle.

__crash 'n burn__ - Any unusually gruesome mountain bike crash. See "dab","faceplant","hammered","groin plant" etc.

__dab__ - To inadvertantly touch the ground with any portion of one's anatomy while negotiating a trail. Variations include foot dab, face dab, body dab, head dab, etc.

__deadpoint__ - point of weightlessness reached after a dyno-move.

__derailleur__ ("de-rail-er" down South) rear shifting device that constitutes the Achilles Heel of mountain bike engineering.

__downshift__ - any shift to a lower gear. See "upshift"

__dyno__ - prefix denoting dramatic rider-bike movement. Short for "dynamic". As in "dyno-move", "dyno-turn", etc.

__event horizon__ - maximum sight distance on trail or minimum braking/reaction time to a given obstacle.

__faceplant__ - a face-first crash 'n burn. Head dab.

__fall line__ - the theoretical line denoting the most direct way down a pitch or obstacle. Mountain bikes generally operate best just off the fall line when descending or ascending.

160

<u>fire road</u> (a.k.a. "fire trail") Usually a rustic doubletrack trail intended for vehicular access in the event of forest fires. Excellent riding, generally.

<u>fun hog</u> - Type T Multiple Personality. Obsessively involved in a number of "thrill sports"; mountain biking plus alpine skiing and/or river running and/or rockclimbing, etc.

<u>geek</u> - beginner or particularly inept mountain biker.

<u>gnarly</u> - universal descriptive term indicating terrain that is difficult, technical, steep, and convoluted.

<u>groinplant</u> - to strike part of your bike (seat, top tube, bars, etc) with your groin in a crash or near-crash.

<u>hammered</u> - violent body-slamming crash or the result of riding all day on a super-gnarly trail.

<u>hellride</u> - any particularly bad trail or bad day on a trail. A.k.a "Bataan Death Ride", "Exploratory Ride", "Puke-O-Rama"

<u>helmet</u> - Brain damage prevention device worn by all rational mountain bikers.

<u>hone</u> - polishing a move or series of moves by subtracting extraneous rider movement.

<u>honed</u> - a very adept rider (uncommon usage). Usually an insult describing any adept-but-obnoxiously-egotistical rider.

<u>honking</u> - a pedalling technique whereby the rider uses his/her body weight to rotate the pedals on the downstroke.

<u>legburn</u> - to totally fry one's legs by forcing them to perform an extended period of anaerobic activity. See "blown," "micro-rest".

<u>limbo log</u> - a log or limb suspended over the trail at approximately face level. A.k.a. "sweeper". See "clotheslined".

<u>load</u> - a dynamic weight shift to one or both tires just prior to a hop or dyno-move.

<u>Macro-focus</u> - The art of seeing the whole trail, not just the area immediately in front of your bike. A rider lacking macro-focus tends to porpoise. See "Micro-focus", "porpoising."

<u>magnetic turn</u> - a decreasing radius turn that centrifugally pulls you to the outside of the turn, often off the trail entirely! Usually seen descending tight switchback loops...

161

<u>mechanic</u> - any person who actually knows what he/she is doing when working on a bike. A.k.a. "gear-head", "bike doc", etc. Most of us regular mountain bikers are in actuality "semi-mechanics", and that's on our <u>good</u> days!

<u>micro-focus</u> - to concentrate fully on the small portion of the trail immediately in front of your bike. While micro-focus is useful for timing & executing "peak moves", it's best to see the whole trail in front of you (macro-focus).

<u>micro-rest</u> - A specialized pedalling technique wherein the rider dyno-relaxes his/her leg on the upstroke to allow oxygen to enter and lactic acid/CO_2 to exit leg muscles. Micro-resting converts anaerobic activity to aerobic activity.

<u>organic obstacle</u> - There are two basic types of organic obstacles; ① "fast organic obstacles" - hikers, horses, deer, etc. and ② "slow organic obstacles" - trees, logs, roots, vines, etc. Fast organic obstacles are to be avoided when possible!

<u>peak move</u>(s) - the key "move" a rider must successfully execute to surmount a difficult stretch of trail.

<u>pitch</u> - any notable upgrade or downgrade on a trail.

<u>pivot turn</u> - to spin the bike on one wheel via body torque. Front wheel pivot turns are possible but the rear wheel pivot turn is the style most commonly used ontrail.

<u>porpoising</u> - riding in a reactionary manner; responding to the bike instead of making the bike respond to you.

<u>punch</u> - to dynamically load the handlebars and/or the seat to compress the tire(s) for a hop.

<u>racerhead</u> - one who races mountain bikes. A mild put-down to describe riders so into competition that they've lost their perspective on the cosmic absurdity of mountain biking.

<u>runout</u> - area just below a serious downgrade where you attempt to regain control after a fast descent. The longer the runout, the faster the descent!

<u>singletrack</u> - Mountain Bike Nirvana.. any trail thru the woods too narrow for a jeep.

<u>stance</u> - How the rider physically relates to his/her bike while riding. Your stance largely determines the handling

162

characteristics of your bike ... different stance, different handling characteristics. [See pp 16-21]

<u>toe clips</u> ("chinese toe cuffs", "toe cuffs") Pedal-mounted foot-retention devices. A <u>must</u> for good overall riding technique!

<u>trials</u> - any highly technical trail, section of trail, or set of obstacles. Roughly translated, "trials" means "most difficult". Variations in this book include "trials trail", "trialsesque", "trials-like", etc. Traditional trials riding involves negotiating ridiculous obstacles without "dabbing".

<u>tune up</u> - to periodically inspect and readjust your bike to insure safety and reliability. Until you gain considerable experience in bike mechanics, have a professional do it!

<u>tweaked</u> - a low glancing blow by a rock, root, or stump that unbalances the rider and/or sheers components off the bike (pedals, cranks, derailleur, etc.). Recovering from a good tweak requires instantaneous handlebar torque!

<u>upshift</u> - any shift to a higher gear (see "downshift").

<u>wheelie</u> - to stand the bike up on the rear wheel by pulling up on the handlebars and taking a hard pedal stroke in a relatively low gear.

<u>wheelie hop</u> - a hop wherein the bike takes off front wheel first, followed by the rear wheel. By comparison, when doing a bunny-hop, both wheels leave the ground simultaneously. The wheelie hop is one of the most difficult advanced "moves" in mountain biking.

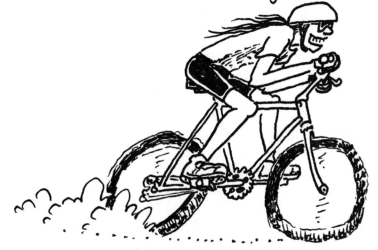